Fat Grafting: Current Concept, Clinical Application, and Regenerative Potential, Part 2

Editors

LEE L.Q. PU
KOTARO YOSHIMURA
SYDNEY R. COLEMAN

CLINICS IN PLASTIC SURGERY

www.plasticsurgery.theclinics.com

July 2015 • Volume 42 • Number 3

ELSEVIER

1600 John F. Kennedy Boulevard ● Suite 1800 ● Philadelphia, Pennsylvania, 19103-2899

http://www.theclinics.com

CLINICS IN PLASTIC SURGERY Volume 42, Number 3
July 2015 ISSN 0094-1298, ISBN-13: 978-0-323-39270-9

Editor: Joanne Husovski
Developmental Editor: Donald Mumford

Clinics in Plastic Surgery (ISSN 0094-1298) is published quarterly by Elsevier Inc., 360 Park Avenue South, New York, NY 10010-1710. Months of issue are January, April, July, and October. Business and Editorial Offices: 1600 John F. Kennedy Blvd., Suite 1800, Philadelphia, PA 19103-2899. Periodicals postage paid at New York, NY and additional mailing offices. Subscription prices are $490.00 per year for US individuals, $716.00 per year for US institutions, $240.00 per year for US students and residents, $555.00 per year for Canadian individuals, $853.00 per year for Canadian institutions, $630.00 per year for international individuals, $853.00 per year for international institutions, and $305.00 per year for Canadian and foreign students/residents. To receive student/resident rate, orders must be accompanied by name of affiliated institution, date of term, and the *signature* of program/residency coordinator on institution letterhead. Orders will be billed at individual rate until proof of status is received. Foreign air speed delivery is included in all *Clinics* subscription prices. All prices are subject to change without notice. **POSTMASTER:** Send address changes to *Clinics in Plastic Surgery*, Elsevier Health Sciences Division, Subscription Customer Service, 3251 Riverport Lane, Maryland Heights, MO 63043. **Customer Service: 1-800-654-2452 (US and Canada). From outside of the United States and Canada, call 314-447-8871. Fax: 314-447-8029. E-mail: JournalsCustomerService-usa@elsevier.com (for print support); JournalsOnlineSupport-usa@elsevier.com (for online support).**

Reprints. For copies of 100 or more of articles in this publication, please contact the Commercial Reprints Department, Elsevier Inc., 360 Park Avenue South, New York, New York 10010-1710. Tel.: +1-212-633-3874; Fax: +1-212-633-3820; E-mail: reprints@elsevier.com.

Clinics in Plastic Surgery is covered in *Current Contents, EMBASE/Excerpta Medica, Science Citation Index, MEDLINE/ PubMed (Index Medicus), ASCA,* and *ISI/BIOMED.*

Contributors

EDITORS

LEE L.Q. PU, MD, PhD, FACS
Professor, Division of Plastic Surgery,
University of California, Davis, Sacramento,
California

KOTARO YOSHIMURA, MD
Associate Professor, Department of Plastic
Surgery, School of Medicine, University of
Tokyo, Bunkyo-Ku, Tokyo, Japan

SYDNEY R. COLEMAN, MD
Clinical Assistant Professor of Plastic Surgery,
New York University, New York, New York;
University of Pittsburgh, Pittsburgh,
Pennsylvania

AUTHORS

NAMRATA ANAVEKAR, FRACS
Plastic Surgery Fellow, Clinique Nescens Paris
Spontini, Paris, France

ERIC AUCLAIR, MD
Private Practice, Paris, France

VALERIA BANDI, MD
Plastic Surgery Unit, Department of Medical
Biotechnology and Translational Medicine
BIOMETRA, Humanitas Clinical and Research
Center, Reconstructive and Aesthetic Plastic
Surgery School, University of Milan, Milan, Italy

BARBARA BANZATTI, MD
Plastic Surgery Unit, Department of Medical
Biotechnology and Translational Medicine
BIOMETRA, Humanitas Clinical and Research
Center, Reconstructive and Aesthetic Plastic
Surgery School, University of Milan, Milan, Italy

DJIAZI BENYAHI, MD
Institut du Sein, Paris, France

FRANCESCO BERTOLINI, MD, PhD
Division of Laboratory Haematology-Oncology,
European Institute of Oncology, Milan, Italy

GIOVANNA CANTARELLA, MD
Department of Otolaryngology, Fondazione
Ospedale Maggiore Policlinico, Ca' Granda,
IRCCS, Milano, Italy

BARBARA CATANIA, MD
Plastic Surgery Unit, Department of Medical
Biotechnology and Translational Medicine
BIOMETRA, Humanitas Clinical and Research
Center, Reconstructive and Aesthetic Plastic
Surgery School, University of Milan, Milan, Italy

FABIO CAVIGGIOLI, MD
Plastic Surgery Unit, Reconstructive and
Aesthetic Plastic Surgery School, MultiMedica
Holding S.p.A., University of Milan, Milan, Italy

KRISHNA BENTLEY CLOUGH, MD
Institut du Sein, Paris, France

SYDNEY R. COLEMAN, MD
Clinical Assistant Professor of Plastic Surgery,
New York University, New York, New York;
University of Pittsburgh, Pittsburgh,
Pennsylvania

AURÉLIE DAUMAS, MD
Internal Medicine Department, Assistance
Publique Hôpitaux de Marseilles (AP-HM),
Aix-Marseilles University, Marseilles, France

EMMANUEL DELAY, MD, PhD
Head of Plastic and Reconstructive Surgery
Department (University Lyon1), Léon Bérard
Center; Private Practice, Lyon, France

DAVIDE FORCELLINI, MD
Plastic Surgery Unit, Reconstructive and
Aesthetic Plastic Surgery School,
MultiMedica Holding S.p.A., University of
Milan, Milan, Italy

KATHERINE LOUISE GALE, MD
Division of Oncoplastic Surgery, Waitemata
DHB, Auckland, New Zealand

SILVIA GIANNASI, MD
Plastic Surgery Unit, Department of Medical
Biotechnology and Translational Medicine
BIOMETRA, Humanitas Clinical and Research
Center, Reconstructive and Aesthetic Plastic
Surgery School, University of Milan, Milan,
Italy

BRIGITTE GRANEL, MD
Internal Medicine Department, Assistance
Publique Hôpitaux de Marseilles (AP-HM);
Vascular Research Center Marseilles, INSERM
UMRS-1076, Aix-Marseilles University,
Marseilles, France

SAMIA GUERID, MD
Plastic and Reconstructive Surgery
Department (University Lyon1), Léon Bérard
Center, Lyon, France

STEVEN E.R. HOVIUS, MD, PhD
Department of Plastic and Reconstructive
Surgery, Erasmus University Medical Center,
Rotterdam, The Netherlands

HESTER J. KAN, MD
Department of Plastic and Reconstructive
Surgery, Erasmus University Medical Center,
Rotterdam, The Netherlands

EVAN B. KATZEL, MD
Department of Plastic Surgery, University of
Pittsburgh Medical Center, Pittsburgh,
Pennsylvania

ROGER K. KHOURI, MD, FACS
Miami Hand Center, Miami, Florida; Miami
Breast Center, Key Biscayne, Florida

FRANCESCO KLINGER, MD
Plastic Surgery Unit, Reconstructive and
Aesthetic Plastic Surgery School,
MultiMedica Holding S.p.A., University of
Milan, Milan, Italy

MARCO KLINGER, MD
Professor, Plastic Surgery Unit, Department
of Medical Biotechnology and Translational
Medicine BIOMETRA, Humanitas Clinical
and Research Center, Reconstructive and
Aesthetic Plastic Surgery School, University
of Milan, Milan, Italy

TOMASZ R. KOSOWSKI, MD
Miami Breast Center, Key Biscayne, Florida

ANDREA LISA, MD
Plastic Surgery Unit, Department of Medical
Biotechnology and Translational Medicine
BIOMETRA, Humanitas Clinical and Research
Center, Reconstructive and Aesthetic Plastic
Surgery School, University of Milan, Milan,
Italy

ROBERT DOUGLAS MACMILLAN, MD, PhD
Division of Oncoplastic Surgery, Nottingham
Breast Institute, Nottingham, United Kingdom

GUY MAGALON, MD
Plastic Surgery Department; Culture and Cell
Therapy Laboratory, INSERM CBT-1409,
Assistance Publique Hôpitaux de Marseilles
(AP-HM), Aix-Marseilles University, Marseilles,
France

JÉRÉMY MAGALON, PharmD
Culture and Cell Therapy Laboratory, INSERM
CBT-1409, Assistance Publique Hôpitaux de
Marseilles (AP-HM), Aix-Marseilles University,
Marseilles, France

LUCA MAIONE, MD
Plastic Surgery Unit, Department of Medical
Biotechnology and Translational Medicine
BIOMETRA, Humanitas Clinical and Research
Center, Reconstructive and Aesthetic Plastic
Surgery School, University of Milan, Milan,
Italy

PATRICK MAISONNEUVE, Eng
Division of Epidemiology and Biostatistics,
European Institute of Oncology, Milan, Italy

ISABELLA C. MAZZOLA, MD
Plastic Surgeon, Department of
Otolaryngology, Fondazione Ospedale
Maggiore Policlinico, Ca' Granda, IRCCS,
Milano, Italy

RICCARDO F. MAZZOLA, MD
Consultant Plastic Surgeon, Department of
Clinical Sciences and Community Health,
Fondazione Ospedale Maggiore Policlinico,
Ca' Granda, IRCCS, Milano, Italy

JEAN YVES PETIT, MD
Division of Plastic and Reconstructive Surgery,
European Institute of Oncology, Milan, Italy

LEE L.Q. PU, MD, PhD, FACS
Professor, Division of Plastic Surgery,
University of California, Davis, Sacramento,
California

PIERRE REY, MD
Division of Plastic and Reconstructive Surgery,
European Institute of Oncology, Milan, Italy;
Centro di Senologia, Genolier Swiss Medical
Network, Lugano, Switzerland

MARIO RIETJENS, MD
Division of Plastic and Reconstructive Surgery,
European Institute of Oncology, Milan, Italy

GINO RIGOTTI, MD
Clinica San Clemente, Mantava, Italy

NICOLE ROTMENSZ, MSc
Director of the Quality Control Unit; Division of
Epidemiology and Biostatistics, European
Institute of Oncology, Milan, Italy

FLORENCE SABATIER, PharmD, PhD
Culture and Cell Therapy Laboratory,
INSERM CBT-1409, Assistance Publique
Hôpitaux de Marseilles (AP-HM); Vascular
Research Center Marseilles, INSERM
UMRS-1076, Aix-Marseilles University,
Marseilles, France

ALESIA P. SABOEIRO, MD
Private Practice, Tribeca Plastic Surgery,
New York, New York

ISABELLE SARFATI, MD
Institut du Sein, Paris, France

NOLWENN SAUTEREAU, MD
Internal Medicine Department, Assistance
Publique Hôpitaux de Marseilles (AP-HM),
Aix-Marseilles University, Marseilles,
France

JENNIFER S.N. VERHOEKX, MD, PhD
Department of Plastic and Reconstructive
Surgery, Erasmus University Medical Center,
Rotterdam, The Netherlands

ALESSANDRA VERONESI, MD
Plastic Surgery Unit, Department of Medical
Biotechnology and Translational Medicine
BIOMETRA, Humanitas Clinical and Research
Center, Reconstructive and Aesthetic Plastic
Surgery School, University of Milan, Milan,
Italy

VALERIANO VINCI, MD
Plastic Surgery Unit, Department of Medical
Biotechnology and Translational Medicine
BIOMETRA, Humanitas Clinical and Research
Center, Reconstructive and Aesthetic Plastic
Surgery School, University of Milan, Milan,
Italy

KOTARO YOSHIMURA, MD
Associate Professor, Department of Plastic
Surgery, School of Medicine, University of
Tokyo, Bunkyo-Ku, Tokyo, Japan

RICCARDO F. MAZZOLA, MD
Consultant Plastic Surgeon, Department of Clinical Sciences and Community Health, Fondazione Ospedale Maggiore Policlinico, Ca Granda, IRCCS, Milano, Italy

JEAN YVES PETIT, MD
Division of Plastic and Reconstructive Surgery, European Institute of Oncology, Milan, Italy

LEE L.Q. PU, MD, PhD, FACS
Professor, Division of Plastic Surgery, University of California, Davis, Sacramento, California

PIERRE REY, MD
Division of Plastic and Reconstructive Surgery, European Institute of Oncology, Milan, Italy; Centro di Senologia, Genolier Swiss Medical Network, Lugano, Switzerland

MARIO RIETJENS, MD
Division of Plastic and Reconstructive Surgery, European Institute of Oncology, Milan, Italy

GINO RIGOTTI, MD
Clinica San Clemente, Mantova, Italy

NICOLE ROTMENSZ, MSc
Director of the Quality Control Unit, Division of Epidemiology and Biostatistics, European Institute of Oncology, Milan, Italy

FLORENCE SABATIER, PharmD, PhD
Culture and Cell Therapy Laboratory, INSERM CBT-1409, Assistance Publique Hopitaux de Marseilles (AP-HM) Vascular Research Center Marseilles, INSERM UMRS-1076 Aix-Marseilles University, Marseilles, France

ALESIA P. SABOEIRO, MD
Private Practice, Tribeca Plastic Surgery, New York, New York

ISABELLE SARFATI, MD
Institut du Sein, Paris, France

NOLWENN GAUTHERAU, MD
Internal Medicine Department, Assistance Publique Hôpitaux de Marseilles (AP-HM) Aix Marseilles University, Marseilles, France

JENNIFER E.N. VERHOEKX, MD, PhD
Department of Plastic and Reconstructive Surgery, Erasmus University, Medical Center, Rotterdam, The Netherlands

ALESSANDRA VERONESI, MD
Plastic Surgery Unit, Department of Medical Biotechnology and Translational Medicine BIOMETRA, Humanitas Clinical and Research Center, Reconstructive and Aesthetic Plastic Surgery School, University of Milan, Milan, Italy

VALERIANO VINCI, MD
Plastic Surgery Unit, Department of Medical Biotechnology and Translational Medicine BIOMETRA, Humanitas Clinical and Research Center, Reconstructive and Aesthetic Plastic Surgery School, University of Milan, Milan, Italy

KOTARO YOSHIMURA, MD
Associate Professor, Department of Plastic Surgery, School of Medicine, University of Tokyo, Bunkyo-ku, Tokyo, Japan

Contents

> Plastic surgeons have come to realize that fat grafting can rejuvenate an aging face by restoring or creating fullness. However, fat grafting does much more than simply add volume. Grafted fat can transform or repair the tissues into which it is placed. Historically, surgeons have hesitated to embrace the rejuvenating potential of fat grafting because of poor graft take, fat necrosis, and inconsistent outcomes. This article describes fat grafting techniques and practices to assist readers in successful harvesting, processing, and placement of fat for optimal graft retention and facial esthetic outcomes.

> The controversy over fat grafting to the breasts has now been settled. In 2009, the American Society of Plastic Surgeons Fat Graft Task Force stated that "Fat grafting may be considered for breast augmentation and correction of defects associated with medical conditions and previous breast surgeries; however, results are dependent on technique and surgeon expertise." This article discusses the history, indications, planning, complications, and present technique of fat grafting to the breast using the Coleman technique.

> Composite breast augmentation is a simple procedure combining the ability of an implant to provide increased volume with the reshaping possibilities offered by fat grafting. The ability to camouflage the implant allows use of a premuscular, retrofascial pocket, avoiding the disadvantages and morbidity associated with retromuscular positioning.

> Breast lipomodeling, or breast fat grafting, is a major development in breast plastic surgery. This technique has a low complication rate, excellent results, and patient acceptance. Radiologic evaluation mostly shows a normal-appearing breast. During breast reconstruction, fat grafting is the ideal complement of the latissimus dorsi flap. Fat grafting for Poland syndrome seems to be a great step and will most likely drastically change the surgical treatment of severe cases. Finally, lipomodeling is a new alternative in the treatment of pectus excavatum, tuberous breasts, and breast asymmetries.

endothelial progenitors, and immune cells. Fat grafting is being increasingly applied in autoimmune diseases, and this article focuses on systemic sclerosis, a rare autoimmune disease characterized by skin fibrosis and microvascular damage. The authors' approach of using fat graft in the face and adipose-tissue-derived stromal vascular fraction for hands is presented as innovative and promising therapy for patients with systemic sclerosis.

 Videonasoendoscopy pre-operative and post-operative of fat injection in a patient affected by velopharyngeal insufficiency accompanies this article

Surgical management of velopharyngeal incompetence (VPI) aims at improving voice resonance and correcting nasal air escape by restoring a competent velopharyngeal sphincter. Assessment of VPI requires the examination of multiple variables. The dynamic study of movements of the velopharyngeal port during speech and the quantification of the closure gap, using flexible videonasoendoscopy and/or videofluoroscopy, is essential. Autologous fat injection represents a minimally invasive alternative to major surgery in the management of mild to moderate VPI that minimizes the risk of complications and sequelae, and can be performed without modifying the anatomy of the velopharyngeal port.

Dupuytren disease is a progressive fibroproliferative disorder, which leads to flexion contractures of the digits. A minimally invasive technique consisting of an extensive percutaneous aponeurotomy of the cord with a needle combined with lipofilling is presented. The selective cutting of the cords under continuous tension disintegrates the cords while sparing the looser neurovascular bundles. Subsequently, lipoaspirate is injected subcutaneously. The authors' prospective results show a significantly shorter recovery time and less overall complications in this technique when compared with open surgery, while no significant difference was observed in the extent of immediate contracture correction and in the recurrence rate at 1 year follow-up.

Recent technical and scientific advances in fat grafting procedures and concepts have improved predictability of fat grafting. Large-volume fat injection is gaining much attention as an attracting procedure for body contouring and reconstruction, but an increasing number of complications also has been recognized over the world. In this article, typical complications after fat grafting are described, as well as an explanation of how and why they occur, and how surgeons can avoid and treat complications.

Autologous fat grafting is an exciting part of plastic and reconstructive surgery. Fat serves as a filler and its role in tissue regeneration will likely play a more important role in our specialty. As we learn more about the basic science of fat grafting and the standardized techniques and instruments used for fat grafting, this procedure alone or in conjunction with invasive procedures may be able to replace many operations that we perform currently. Its minimally invasive nature will benefit greatly our cosmetic and reconstructive patients, and may even achieve better clinical outcomes.

CLINICS IN PLASTIC SURGERY

ISSUE OF RELATED INTEREST

Midface and Periocular Rejuvenation
Editor: Anthony P. Sclafani
Facial Plastic Surgery Clinics
May 2015. Volume 23, Issue 2
Available at: http://www.facialplastic.theclinics.com/

THE CLINICS ARE AVAILABLE ONLINE!
Access your subscription at:
www.theclinics.com

CLINICS IN PLASTIC SURGERY

Preface
Fat Grafting: Current Concept, Clinical Application, and Regenerative Potential, Part 2

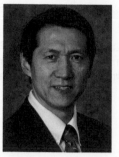
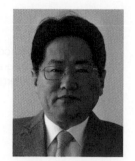
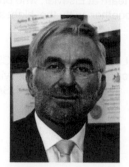

Lee L.Q. Pu, MD, PhD, FACS   Kotaro Yoshimura, MD   Sydney R. Coleman, MD

Editors

Although fat grafting had a "bad reputation" in the past, it has become one of the most commonly performed procedures in both aesthetic and reconstructive plastic surgery. It started as autologous filler for facial rejuvenation, but now it has been used not only for facial rejuvenation but also for breast surgery, body contouring surgery, and other aspects of aesthetic and reconstructive surgery. Until recently, fat grafting has showed its regenerative potential and has been used to treat some of the difficult clinical problems facing plastic surgeons. As we know more about fat grafting, its mechanisms of how fat grafts survive, and their regenerative features, fat grafting as a relatively noninvasive procedure can gradually replace many aesthetic and reconstructive procedures in the future. It becomes a major armamentarium for plastic surgeons to rejuvenate aged tissues, to reconstruct a missing part of tissues, to reverse the disease process, and to treat certain pathologic conditions.

Because fat grafting has become a rapidly growing field in plastic surgery with much new advancement for aesthetic and reconstructive surgery, several visionary leaders, including the three editors of this issue, have formed a brand new international society, named International Society of Plastic and Regenerative Surgery

(ISPRES), in 2011. This young, dynamic international society has gathered many talented plastic surgeons with primary interests and expertise in fat grafting. This issue and the April 2015 issue of *Clinics in Plastic Surgery* represent members of this young international organization and their excellent work being presented during the previous world congresses in Rome, Italy, Berlin, Germany, and Miami, USA. Part II starts with fat grafting for facial filling and regeneration followed by fat grafting for primary breast augmentation and composite breast augmentation with an implant and fat grafts. The role of fat grafting in breast reconstruction and breast reconstruction with fat grafting and Brava are well presented in this issue. This is followed by the best summary on safety considerations of fat grafting to the breast. Fat grafting as a regenerative approach to a number of difficult clinical programs, such as chronic ulcer or scar, scleroderma, velopharyngeal insufficiency, and Dupytren contracture, is also presented in this issue. In the last two articles, management of complications related to fat grafting and future perspective of fat grafting is included for the completion of this special issue.

We sincerely hope that you will enjoy reading this special issue of *Clinics in Plastic Surgery*. It represents a true team effort from worldwide

Clin Plastic Surg 42 (2015) xiii–xiv
http://dx.doi.org/10.1016/j.cps.2015.05.001
0094-1298/15/$ – see front matter © 2015 Published by Elsevier Inc.

experts of the ISPRES. We would like to express our heartfelt gratitude to all of the contributors for their expertise, dedication, and responsibility to produce such a world class issue of plastic surgery. It is certainly our privilege to work with these respected authors in this exciting field of plastic surgery. We would also like to express our appreciation to the publication team at Elsevier, who put this remarkable issue together with the highest possible standard.

Lee L.Q. Pu, MD, PhD, FACS
University of California, Davis
Sacramento, CA, USA

Kotaro Yoshimura, MD
University of Tokyo
Tokyo, Japan

Sydney R. Coleman, MD
New York University
New York, NY, USA

University of Pittsburgh
Pittsburgh, PA, USA

E-mail addresses:
lee.pu@ucdmc.ucdavis.edu (L.L.Q. Pu)
kotaro-yoshimura@umin.ac.jp (K. Yoshimura)
sydcoleman@me.com (S.R. Coleman)

Fat Grafting for Facial Filling and Regeneration

Sydney R. Coleman, MD[a],*, Evan B. Katzel, MD[b]

KEYWORDS

- Fat grafting • Structural fat grafting • Coleman technique • Facial augmentation • Autologous fat
- Fat • Lipoaspirate • Adipose-derived stem cells

KEY POINTS

- Fat grafting is a well-established technique to restore volume and enhance the quality of skin in the aging face.
- Harvesting by hand using 10-mL syringes is recommended to avoid traumatizing fat.
- Sterile centrifugation at 1286g for 2 minutes should be used for processing.
- Blunt tip cannulas should be used to diffusely transplant fat and avoid intravascular injection.
- Fat should be infused in small aliquots no greater than 0.1 mL per pass to encourage proximity to a blood supply and avoid fat resorption, necrosis, or oil cyst formation.
- Varying the depth of fat injection brings about desired cosmetic results.
- Maximal graft retention results from adherence to precise technique.
- Improvements in the quality of the overlying skin can be quite dramatic.

INTRODUCTION

The key to fat grafting in the face is to appreciate and use the ability of fat to transform and rejuvenate the tissues into which it is placed. The first attempts of fat grafting to the face were performed to not only restore fullness but also improve the quality of the tissue into which the fat was grafted, including scars. In 1893, Gustav Neuber[1] described the use of transplanted fat not only for filling but also the reconstruction of an ugly depressed facial scar. Even in this earliest description of fat grafting, the surgeon recognized the importance of the transformation of the tissues into which the fat was placed. In this first reported case, the grafted fat was noted to improve the scarring.

Holländer[2] was the first to describe a technique for the injection of fat using a cannula in 1909. After 3 years, in 1912, he published more extensive descriptions of the injection technique and photographs of his results, in which he not only restored fullness to facial atrophy but also described the correction of adherent scars and adhesions and improvement in the tissues into which the grafted fat was injected.[3]

With the arrival of liposuction in the early 1980s, plastic surgeons had a new source for soft tissue filler, the lipoaspirate from liposuction.

Unfortunately, the surgeons in the 1980s who first used fat grafting implanted the grafts into the face with a bolus technique, which had less-than-desirable reported results.[4,5] In these reports, the surgeons described resorption of the fat without any other changes.

In the early 1990s, Coleman[6–8] introduced the technique of processing the fat by centrifuging

Disclosures: Royalties for instruments sold by Mentor, paid consultant for Armed Forces Institute of Regenerative Medicine, paid consultant for Mentor Worldwide LLC, paid consultant for Musculoskeletal Transplant Foundation, and paid Consultant for LifeCell (S.R. Coleman); No disclosures (E.B. Katzel).
[a] Department of Plastic Surgery, New York University Langone Medical Center, New York, NY, USA;
[b] Department of Plastic Surgery, University of Pittsburgh Medical Center, Pittsburgh, PA, USA
* Corresponding author.
E-mail address: lipostructure@yahoo.com

and separating out the unwanted components (oil, blood, local anesthetic, and other noncellular material) and placing the fat in tiny aliquots with each pass of the cannula. Placement of the fat in small aliquots ensured the proximity of the injected fat to a blood supply and anchored the fat into the recipient tissue. This technique has been given many names, such as structural fat grafting, Lipo-Structure®, or the Coleman technique.

With more reliable techniques and instrumentation, fat grafting and harvesting and injecting with cannulas gradually become more popular. As a result, attention has returned to approaching facial rejuvenation not only by cutting and lifting but also through the restoration of fullness.

During this resurgence of fat grafting for the correction of atrophy associated with aging, an exciting observation has been made by the surgeons placing fat under sun-damaged, aging, and scarred skin. There has been a transformation of the skin over time. The change observed is an improvement in the texture of the overlying skin, which includes one or all of the following: a decrease in wrinkling, a decrease in the size of pores, an improvement in skin color, an apparent thickening of the skin, an improvement in facial scarring, and a smoother, younger appearance.

In this article, the details of the Coleman technique, including harvesting, refinement, and placement methods are described to aid practitioners in obtaining long-term, consistent, and esthetically pleasing results for facial rejuvenation.[6,7] Patient selection and indications for facial fat grafting, potential complications, postoperative care, and current and future research and trends will be discussed (**Table 1**).

Table 1
Current research on fat grafting

Title	Author	Journal	Summary
"Grading Lipoaspirate: Is There an Optimal Density for Fat Grafting?"	Allen et al,[9] 2013	*Plastic and Reconstructive Surgery*	More of the highest-density fractions of lipoaspirate were preserved over time compared with lower-density fractions. High-density fractions contained more progenitor cells and larger concentrations of several vasculogenic mediators compared with the lower-density fractions
"Endogenous Stem Cell Therapy Enhances Fat Graft Survival"	Butala et al,[10] 2012	*Plastic and Reconstructive Surgery*	Endogenous progenitor cell mobilization enhanced low-density fat neovascularization, increased vasculogenic cytokine expression, and improved graft survival to a level equal to that of high-density fat grafts
"Double-Blind Clinical Trial to Compare Autologous Fat Grafts Versus Autologous Fat Grafts with PDGF: No Effect of PDGF"	Fontdevila et al,[11] 2014	*Plastic and Reconstructive Surgery*	The addition of plasma-rich growth factors to the adipose tissue graft did not improve outcomes
"Prevalence of Endogenous CD34+ Adipose Stem Cells Predicts Human Fat Graft Retention in a Xenograft Model"	Philips et al,[12] 2012	*Plastic and Reconstructive Surgery*	Concentration of CD34+ progenitor cells within the stromal vascular fraction may be used to predict human fat graft retention
"Application of Platelet-Rich Plasma and Platelet-Rich Fibrin in Fat Grafting: Basic Science and Literature Review"	Liao et al	*Tissue Engineering Part B Reviews*	This article provides a general foundation on which to critically evaluate earlier studies, discuss the limitations of previous research, and direct plans for future experiments to improve the optimal effects of platelet-rich plasma in fat grafting

TREATMENT GOALS AND PLANNED OUTCOMES

The first step in facial rejuvenation is identifying the patient's complaints and goals. The next step is a thorough analysis of the face, donor sites, and general patient selection criteria.[13] Fat grafting can be a tremendous tool for facial rejuvenation; however, in the excessively sagging face with redundant loose skin, fat grafting alone may not give the patient an adequate change. The face should be analyzed in a systematic manner to assess the needs of each potential patient. In the youthful face, the skin of the forehead is tight and free of rhytids and the brow and glabella are unfurrowed. The upper eyelids and orbits are full. The cheeks are full and rounded with the fat pad hiding the zygomatic arch. The buccal cheek may have a slight hollowing but only appears gaunt in the thinnest patients. The nasolabial folds are soft and the lips full, pouted, and averted, with the lower lip slightly larger than the upper lip. The jaw line is sharp, with a well-defined chin.

As a person progresses toward middle age, lines and folds become apparent on the forehead and glabella. The temples begin to hollow, as do the orbits. As the upper eyelid loses fullness, the skin of the upper lid empties out. This process can result in sagging of the excess skin, or the skin can retreat into the orbit giving a hollow appearance.[14] The lid-cheek junction elongates, because the inferior orbital rim becomes more prominent again because of volume loss. The tear trough deepens, as do the nasolabial and marionette folds. The zygomatic arch becomes more apparent as the malar fat pads deflate and the border of the mandible weakens with atrophy and becomes less defined because of relative ascent of the posterior and anterior jawline concomitantly with the descent of the jowl, often with the appearance of excess jowls.[15] These changes become more apparent as aging continues.

Facial fat grafting reverses these changes by restoring volume and appropriate proportions to the face.[16] Unlike traditional temporary fillers, fat has the potential for permanence and improving the quality of the overlying skin and repairing skin damage, thereby rejuvenating the face.[12,17]

In the upper third of the face, forehead and glabellar rhytids can be smoothed and eliminated with both intradermal and superficial fat grafting. Orbital hollowing can be filled with well-placed fat, either alone or in combination with excision of the skin of the upper eyelid.[6] The lower lid and the lid/cheek junction can be returned to a soft, full, youthful appearance with autologous fat augmentation; however, care should be taken to avoid complications in the lower lid.[18] The tear trough deformity can also be reconstructed with carefully placed fat injections, while coverage of the zygomatic arch can be accomplished as well. The lips can be augmented with fat to restore the full, pouty look of youth, while a weak jawline can be corrected with fat grafting along the mandibular border.[19] Finally, fat grafting is extremely valuable in correcting congenital and acquired soft tissue defects of the face, including HIV-related lipoatrophy and Perry-Romberg syndrome, linear scleroderma, surgical defects, and scarring and traumatic loss of soft tissue, as well as underlying bony injuries.[20–23] Similar to the goals in the esthetic patient, fat grafting in the reconstructive realm aims to restore healthy, natural facial contours.

PREOPERATIVE PLANNING

As with any procedure in plastic surgery, all candidates should undergo a thorough preoperative history and physical examination. Attention should be paid in the preoperative assessment to a patient or family history of bleeding or clotting disorders, previous miscarriage, and/or deep vein thrombosis or pulmonary embolism. In addition, all patients should be asked about the use of anticoagulants such as warfarin, Lovenox, aspirin, nonsteroidal antiinflammatory drugs, and certain vitamins and supplements known to adversely affect clotting.

Smoking and tobacco use negatively affect graft take. Thus, smoking status should always be documented in the preoperative workup. Although infection is rare with fat grafting, all patients should be asked about a history of methicillin-resistant *Staphylococcus aureus* infections and previous postsurgical infection.

Time should be spent inquiring about all previous surgical procedures, and patients should be asked specifically about previous cosmetic surgeries and noninvasive procedures. Patients may not consider injection of fillers or liposuction or minimally invasive liposculpting procedures relevant and may not initially recount these procedures unless specifically asked. Such procedures can greatly affect the quantity and quality of fat that can be harvested from a donor site. Patients should be questioned about weight changes and plans for future weight gain or loss. Throughout the preoperative assessment, it is important for the surgeon to gauge the mind-set and goals of the patient. Patients with unrealistic goals are more likely than not to turn into unhappy patients postoperatively.

Photographs of both the donor sites and the recipient sites from a wide variety of angles are critical in fat grafting. Photographs provide the surgeon and the patient with a blueprint for planning surgery, and the photos or tracings can be marked accordingly. In this regard, by reviewing preoperative photographs with the patient, previously unrecognized defects and asymmetries may be pointed out and documented in the medical record. In addition, by comparing preoperative photographs to pictures from the patient in his or her 20s or 30s, the patient is better able to identify areas of concern and possible correction.[6] Using this information, all areas of planned augmentation, cannula entry points, and projected size of grafts can be documented on the preoperative photographs to better prepare the patient for postoperative results. Finally, initial photographs provide a way to compare preoperative appearance with postoperative results.

These preoperative conversations and planning sessions are the basis for informed consent. In addition to spending time analyzing photographs, during a consultation, it is also important to prepare the patient for any possible complications before the day of surgery. Surgical plans, desired outcomes, risks, and benefits should be reviewed again the day of surgery to address any last-minute patient concerns.

PATIENT POSITIONING

Donor and recipient sites dictate patient positioning. As there have been no conclusive studies showing reproducible differences in graft survival from different donor sites, donor site selection is determined by patient preference, the amount of fat required, and the amount of fat available at different sites. Generally, for facial fat grafting, the patient is positioned supine. This positioning allows access to the inner thighs, flank, and abdomen.

The donor sites and face are prepared with Betadine.

PROCEDURAL APPROACH

The Coleman technique for fat grafting described here is nearly identical to the technique first described in the early 1990s.[6–8] The keys to the technique remain gentle harvesting of fat to preserve its delicate structure of parcels, refinement through centrifugation to remove nonviable components and concentrate the fat, and delivery of the fat in small aliquots to ensure adequate blood supply and maximize graft take.[6,7,24] Adherence to these principles results in fat graft retention reliably reaching 65%.[25,26]

Harvesting

Depending on patient preference and the volume of fat required, fat can be harvested under either local or general anesthesia. For straight local cases, nerve blocks may be performed. The infiltration solution consists of 0.5% lidocaine with 1:200,000 epinephrine buffered with sodium bicarbonate (or diluted to half the strength to provide a larger volume) infused with a Lamis (or other blunt) infiltration cannula (Mentor Worldwide LLC, Santa Barbara, CA, USA). When intravenous sedation or general anesthesia is required for harvests of larger volumes of fat, the infiltration solution of choice is 0.1% lidocaine with 1:400,000 epinephrine. For either case, the volume of tumescent solution infused should usually be less than the amount of fat to be harvested.

A multihole Coleman harvesting cannula attached to a 10-mL syringe is then used to suction the fat. The plunger of the syringe is pulled back only a few milliliters to create enough vacuum to harvest the fat, while avoiding excessive pressure that could rupture fat cells. Upon completion of the fat harvest, incisions are closed with interrupted sutures.

Refinement and Purification

After each 10-mL syringe is filled, the cannula is disconnected, a Luer-Lock cap (Becton, Dickinson and Company, Franklin Lakes, NJ, USA) is placed, and the plunger is removed. Syringes are then placed in a sterilized centrifuge rotor and spun at 1286*g* for 2 minutes to separate the components of the tissue. This gravitational force has been found to be the most advantageous for condensing the fat to improve long-term viability[27] and concentrate growth factors. The oil on the surface is decanted, and the Luer-Lock cap is then removed, allowing the aqueous layer to be drained from the bottom of the syringe. A Codman neuropad (Codman Neuro, Raynham, MA, USA) or Telfa strip (Telfa Strip, Salem, MA, USA) is then placed in the top of the syringe to wick away the remaining oil. The processed fat is then transferred to 1-mL syringes for placement.

Centrifugation results in graded densities of the fat, and the highest-density fat remains at the bottom of the 10-mL syringes. Studies have shown better graft take for high-density fat compared with low-density fat.[9] Therefore, when transferring fat from the 10-mL to 1-mL injection syringes, the injection syringes should be grouped into high-density, intermediate-density, and low-density groups to allow for more thoughtful placement.

Placement

Incision sites are anesthetized with 0.5% lidocaine with 1:200,000 epinephrine before making stab incisions with a No. 11 blade. A small volume of 0.5% lidocaine with 1:200,000 epinephrine is then infused into graft sites for anesthesia and vasoconstriction. Vasoconstriction reduces the risk of inadvertent intravascular infusion and reduces postoperative bruising.

Decanted oil collected during the fat processing stage can be used when available to lubricate the incision sites during harvesting to avoid friction on the puncture or incision sites.

One of the keys to the success of the Coleman technique is placing the parcels of grafted fat in proximity to an adequate blood supply. In order to create this environment, fat should be placed in small aliquots surrounded by native tissue. These aliquots should be placed as the cannula is withdrawn, and no more than 0.1 mL of fat should be placed with each pass. Transferring fat parcels that are too large results in fat necrosis, fat resorption, oil cysts, or irregularities.[28] If fat is being used to fill or reconstruct a scar, release of adhesions using special instruments or an 18-gauge needle[29,30] should be performed only after the placement of a significant volume of fat into that area.

Different depths of fat placement should be used, depending on the desired effect. Fat placed in the intradermal or subdermal layers affects the skin more to improve wrinkles, and the overall complexion and skin quality.[31] However, at this level, care should be taken to avoid creating superficial irregularities. Fat placed deep against the periosteum can be used to change how the remaining soft tissue envelope drapes over the bony structure of the face. Fat placed in the intermediate subcutaneous layers restores volume to rejuvenate or establish a different facial proportion. Molding of the fat placed at any level should be avoided, because this may lead to fat necrosis and resorption. Upon completion of graft placement, infusion sites are closed with interrupted sutures. A small volume of concentrated fat (approximately 0.2–0.3 mL) is then placed into the closed incisions using a 22-gauge needle; this is done to aid in healing of the incisions.

COMPLICATIONS AND THEIR MANAGEMENT

Proper adherence to the described technique minimizes complications, because facial fat grafting is generally well tolerated. The most common category of complication is minor esthetic irregularities. Such complications can take the form of palpable lumps because of placement that is too superficial or placement of aliquots that are too large resulting in fat necrosis. Fat grafting in thin-skinned areas should be performed cautiously to avoid such complications.[32] These irregularities can be managed by suction lipectomies using the same cannulas used for infusion, by direct open excision, or with Lipodissolve.[18,33]

All patients undergoing fat grafting experience bruising and swelling postoperatively. Pigmentation of the lower eyelids after fat grafting gives the appearance of dark tea shining through the tear trough and can be referred to as tea staining. This problem generally resolves quickly, but may persist for up to several months, or even a year, in some patients as the skin thickens. Although this should be considered an expected outcome rather than a complication, patients should be prepared for bruising that can last up to 3 weeks after fat placement.

Infection after fat grafting is exceedingly rare. Despite the rarity of infections, strict adherence to sterile technique should be practiced while harvesting, processing, and placing grafts to avoid infection and subsequent fat resorption. Oral site infusion and lip augmentation should be performed last, because these sites are contaminated with oral flora despite Betadine preparation. Patients with a history of cold sores should be receiving prophylaxis with acyclovir.

The most feared possible complication of fat grafting is fat embolism from intravascular infusion. This complication is extremely rare and has never been reported with the use of blunt tip Coleman cannulas for placement. The use of an epinephrine-containing solution at the graft site also reduces the possibility of fat emboli.[34]

POSTOPERATIVE CARE

Standard postoperative liposuction garments or compressive dressings are applied to the donor sites to prevent hematoma and seroma formation. For the first 72 hours postoperatively, cool (but not ice-cold) compresses may be applied to the face intermittently to reduce discomfort, bruising, and swelling. Deep massage of the face should be avoided, because it can cause fat migration or necrosis. However, light touch can be performed to encourage lymphatic migration.

OUTCOMES
Patient 1

A 44-year-old woman originally presented with a history of 3 face-lifts, 3 lower-lid blepharoplasties, and 1 upper blepharoplasty performed elsewhere. The last procedure was performed 3 years before presentation. Preoperatively, she complained of hollowing of the orbits, prominent tear troughs, deepening of her nasolabial folds, loss of malar prominence, rhytids at her oral commissures, marionette lines, and loss of definition of her jawline. A total of 200 mL fat was harvested from her knees as well as inner, outer, and anterior parts of thighs using 10-mL syringes and Coleman harvesting cannulas. The fat was processed in the standard manner using the Coleman technique. Refined fat was then placed as follows: into the right temple, 6 mL; left temple, 6 mL; glabella, 1.5 mL; right medial eyelid, 0.5 mL; left medial eyelid, 0.5 mL; right anterior malar fold, 1.5 mL; left anterior malar fold, 1.5 mL; right anterior malar region, 3 mL; left anterior malar region, 4 mL; right lateral malar region, 7 mL; left lateral malar region, 8 mL; right nasolabial fold, 7 mL; left nasolabial fold, 5 mL; right buccal cheek, 6 mL; left buccal cheek, 4 mL; right mandibular jawline, 4 mL; left mandibular jawline, 4 mL; mental groove, 0.5 mL; and submental region feathering down to the cervical mental angle and upper part of the neck, 6 mL. The fat was placed using a combination of Coleman cannulas and 22-gauge needles, but mostly with the type 3 minicannulas.

The patient returned 2 years later pleased with the result but desiring subtle enhancements. A total volume of 40 mL was removed from donor sites, and processed to yield 15 mL of fat. Fat was placed as follows: right temple, 4.7 mL; left temple, 3.5 mL; left side of her nose, 0.6 mL; right nasolabial fold, 1 mL; and left nasolabial fold, 3 mL.

Photographs (**Fig. 1**) show the patient 22 months after her second procedure (middle photo) and 11 years after the second procedure with no other procedures or fillers in the interim. Most areas of the face were infiltrated with fat, but her lips and nose were not infiltrated. Therefore, the nose and lips look much smaller than they actually are. Patient has not only a lasting restoration of fullness in every area of the face infiltrated with fat but also a remarkable improvement in the quality of skin over time.

Patient 2

A 45-year-old woman presented for upper facial rejuvenation (**Fig. 2**). She had a history of a coronal brow lift, 2 upper blepharoplasties, and 1 lower blepharoplasty.

A total of 60 mL of fat was harvested from right and left thighs using blunt Coleman harvesting cannulas. The fat was processed in the standard manner using the Coleman technique. Refined fat was then placed as follows: into the right temple, 4 mL; left temple, 3.5 mL; right upper eyelid, 2.0 mL; left upper eyelid, 2.5 mL; lateral part of eyelids, 1 mL each; right anterior malar fold, 1.5 mL; left anterior malar fold, 2.0 mL; right anterior malar region, 2.5 mL; and left anterior malar region, 3 mL.

She was so delighted at the change in her periorbital region that she returned 3 years later for lower facial rejuvenation with a little more midface rejuvenation.

For the second procedure, a total of 160 mL fat was harvested from right and left thighs using blunt Coleman harvesting cannulas. The fat was processed in the standard manner using the Coleman technique. To create more fullness, 0.6 mL was placed into the right lateral eyelid and 0.9 mL into the left lateral eyelid.

Refined fat was then placed into the anterior malar regions as follows: 2.5 mL into the right and 3.5 mL into the left, feathering up into the lower eyelid; right nasolabial fold, 4.5 mL; left nasolabial fold, 4.9 mL; right anterior mandibular border, 4 mL; left anterior mandibular border, 4 mL; marionette region, 2.6 mL on the right and 3.5 mL on the left; posterior border of the mandible, 12 mL on the right and 13 mL on the left; and finally, 12 mL into the chin.

After 3 years, the patient returned delighted with her results but wanting additional enhancement. She now wanted stronger cheeks, more definition in her chin, and pouty lips with an attempt at softening the upper lip wrinkles. Using the same technique, 90 mL was harvested from the knees and calves. The refined fat was then placed into the following areas: lateral malar cheeks, 3.9 mL on the right and 3.8 mL on the left; nasolabial folds, 3.2 mL on the right and 3 mL on the left; marionettes, 3.5 mL on the right and 3 mL on the left; upper lip wrinkles, 0.9 mL; white roll, 1 mL; philtrum, 1 mL; upper lip body, 1.5 mL; lower lip body, 2.5 mL; chin, 4 mL; and border of the mandible, 4.5 mL on each side. In all the above procedures, fat was placed using a combination of Coleman cannulas and 22-gauge needles, but mostly with the mini-3 cannulas.

Patient 3

A 53-year-old woman presented with remarkable periorbital pigmentation (**Fig. 3**). She had never had any facial procedures, injectables, or Botox. She notes that she had melasma, which has persisted for years. Her primary complaint was that

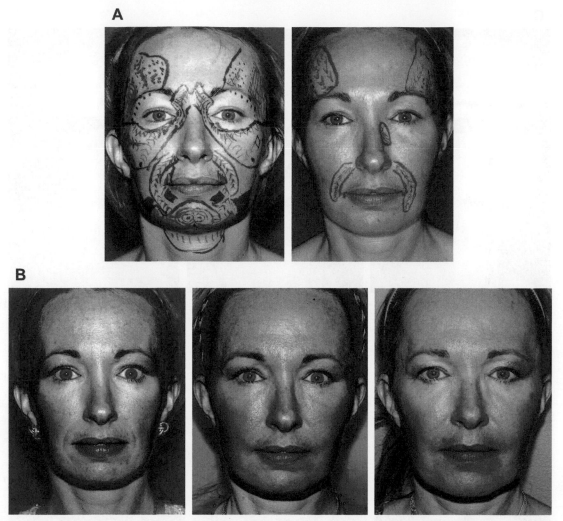

Fig. 1. (*A*) Markings on this 44-year-old patient immediately before the procedure show the extent of the initial fat grafting (*left*). Markings for the next procedure 2 years later (*right*) illustrate the areas of secondary enhancement. The green marks demonstrate changes in shape and size, and the orange borders demonstrate the limits of placement. (*B*) This 44-year-old patient before full-face fat grafting (*left*) 22 months after her second procedure (*center*) previously described. There is a remarkable increase in fullness over the entire face with fat grafting at 22 months. The photo on the right was taken 10 years after her second procedure. There is little change between her 22-month follow-up and her long-term follow-up over 10 years after her last procedure. Please note that the increased fullness of the entire face can be more accurately estimated by the decrease in her relative nose and lip sizes.

she felt her eyelids were hollow and dark so that she looked tired.

A total of 290 mL of fat was harvested from her love handles, medial thighs, and suprapubic area using blunt Coleman harvesting cannulas. The fat was processed in the standard manner using the Coleman technique. The following volumes were placed in her periorbital region: right anterior malar fold, 1.3 mL; left anterior malar fold, 1.3 mL; right lateral eyelid, 0.9 mL; left lateral eyelid, 0.8 mL; right upper eyelid, 1.5 mL; left upper eyelid,

1.5 mL; right medial eye/lateral nose, 0.3 mL; left medial eye/lateral part if the nose, 0.3 mL; right temple, 5.0 mL; left temple, 6.0 mL; forehead transverse wrinkles, 6.0 mL; glabella/nasion, 4.0 mL; right posterior buccal cheek, 3.0 mL; left posterior buccal cheek, 4.0 mL; right malar cheek, 6.0 mL; and left malar cheek, 5.0 mL.

Two years after the initial upper and midface procedures described here, the patient returned delighted with the improvement of her eyelid color and texture wanting to proceed with fat

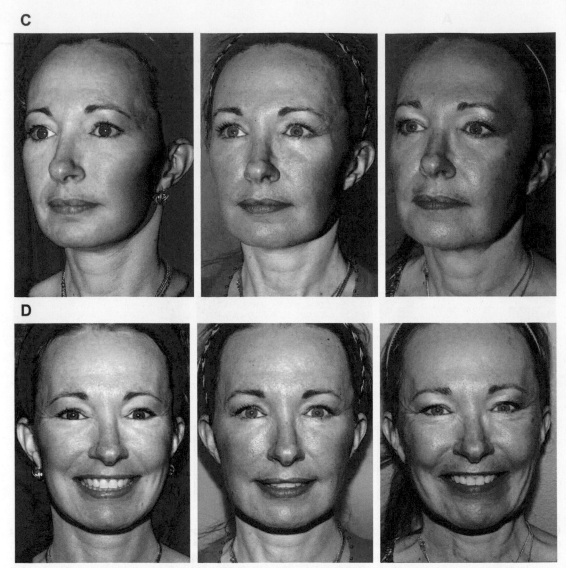

Fig. 1. (*continued*). (*C*) In an oblique view, the same patient before full-face fat grafting (*left*) 22 months after her second procedure (*center*) and over 10 years after her second procedure (*right*). These photos demonstrate the rejuvenating properties of fat grafting throughout the face. Selective increases in fullness over the temples, cheeks, and jaw soften her face. Lowering of the anterior border and posterior border of the mandible can reduce the apparent size of the jowls. Although the fat remains over the 10-year period, some normal aging continues, as can be seen between the 22-month (*middle*) and 10-year (*right*) photos. (*D*) Her face in active motion looks normal.

grafting to the hands and minor enhancements of the periorbital region. For this, 0.9 mL more was placed into the right lower eyelid/cheek and 1.2 mL into the left lower eyelid/cheek; an additional 0.5 mL was placed into the darkest area of her medial eyelid/lateral nose area; and 1 mL more was placed into the glabella/nasion area. In addition, a tiny sliver of skin was removed from the upper eyelid bilaterally to tighten the upper eyelid without removing any fullness.

The patient returned 1 year after her second procedure delighted, saying that she had a "massive improvement" but the change was not detectible to her friends or acquaintances (see **Fig. 1**).

RESULTS

The effect of fat grafting on the face far exceeds the changes in shape and fullness. After fat is placed under the skin, changes begin to take place. Initially, fullness is obvious. Then, gradually,

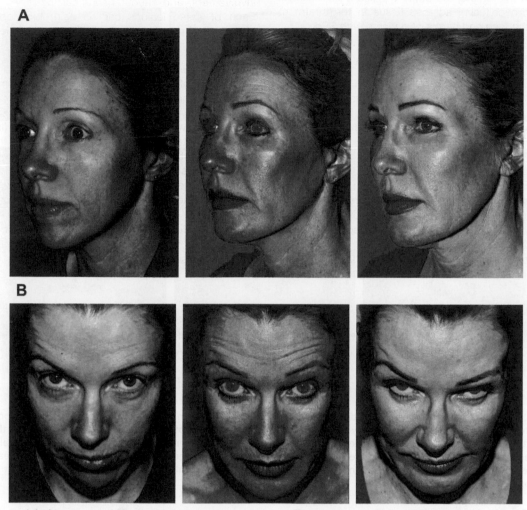

Fig. 2. (*A*) This 45-year-old patient had a staged approach to fat grafting starting with periorbital grafting, and then lower facial fat grafting 3 years later (*left*). The middle photograph is 3 years after her lower facial fat grafting at which time she had minor enhancements primarily to her lateral malar and periorbital regions. She is shown 4 years after the procedure (*right*). (*B*) The patient is shown before (*left*), 3 years after the first 2 procedures (*middle*), and then 4 years after the third procedure (*right*). The effect of adjusting facial proportion is demonstrated by the enlargement of the cheeks to suppress the lower lid fat pads.

over the following months, changes in the skin are noted. There is a reduction of wrinkles and crepiness, which is accompanied by an apparent thickening of the skin and a softening or even elimination of scars. Over a longer period, up to a year or more, there is an improvement in the color of the skin. These changes result in what appears to be a repair of aging or sun-damaged skin.

DISCUSSION

The key to successful structural fat grafting to the face is to understand how to place fat in different levels and to use the graded densities in fat to accomplish maximal predictability. The placement of similar densities of fat into bilateral areas helps to avoid potential uneven fullness or changes in the overlying skin.

In the face, the use of smaller-bore cannulas for placement gives surgeons greater control, which allows them to be more precise. The cannulas used in the perioral, periorbital, and nasal area are 17 gauge or smaller in diameter.

The use of additives such as stromal vascular fraction and growth factors such as platelet-rich plasma may increase the predictability of fat grafting, but definitive studies have yet to become available.

C

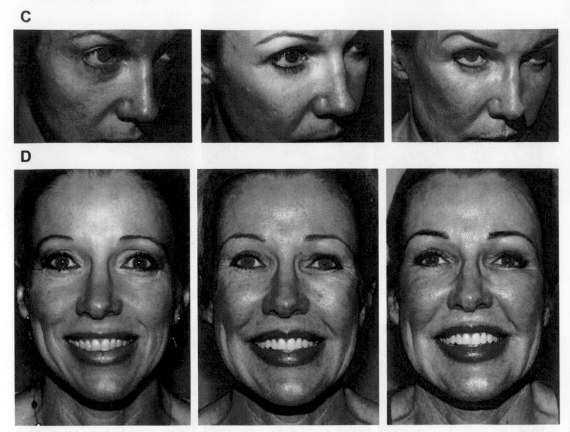

D

Fig. 2. (*continued*). (*C*) Again the patient is shown before any fat grafting (*top*), 3 years after the first 2 procedures (*middle*), and then another 4 years after the third procedure (*bottom*). Please note the change in the texture of the skin, as well as the decrease in pore size. Between the lower 2 photos, augmentation of the malar cheek laterally is obvious. (*D*) The patient before (*left*), 3 years after the second fat grafting (*middle*), and 4 years after the third fat grafting. Note the natural appearance with the patient smiling, as well as the adjustment of proportion more obvious in this view.

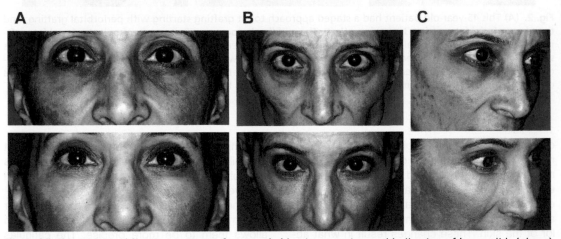

Fig. 3. (*A*) This 53-year-old patient presents for remarkable pigmentation and hollowing of her eyelids (*above*). She had fat grafted over her lower eyelids, cheeks, temples, nasion, and glabella and had excision of upper eyelid skin. One year after her last procedure (*below*), she has not only an improvement in color of her eyelids but also a remarkable improvement in eyelid and cheek texture with remarkable improvement in the pore size. (*B*) This view demonstrates not only the remarkable improvement in color and texture but also a subtle change in the fullness of her cheeks, temples, and nasion/glabella. (*C*) This view is particularly helpful to visualize the improvement in the quality and color of skin after fat grafting, especially in the medial eyelid/lateral nose 1 year after the last fat grafting to the area.

SUMMARY

The goal of this article was to share proven techniques for harvesting, processing, and placing fat in order to allow surgeons to provide the best, most reproducible outcomes with autologous fat grafting in the face.

Fat grafting outcomes can vary greatly based on the technique. Over the past 25 years, few advances have been made in fat grafting. However, in the near future, research and refinements in instrumentation and techniques will probably lead to more predictable outcomes.

REFERENCES

1. Neuber G. Fettransplantation. Bericht Uber die Verhandlungen der Deutschen Gesellschaft fur Chirurgie. Zbl Chir 1893;30:66.
2. Holländer E. Berliner klinischer Wochenschrift. 1909;18.
3. Holländer E. Die kosmetische Chirurgie (S.669-712, 45 Abb.). In: Joseph M, editor. Handbuch der kosmetik. Leipzig (Germany): Verlag van Veit & co; 1912. p. 690–1.
4. Ellenbogen R. Autologous fat injection. Plast Reconstr Surg 1991;88(3):543–4.
5. Ersek RA. Transplantation of purified autologous fat: a 3-year follow-up is disappointing. Plast Reconstr Surg 1991;87(2):219–27.
6. Coleman SR. The technique of periorbital lipoinflitration. Operat Tech Plast Reconstr Surg 1994;1(3): 120–6.
7. Coleman SR. Long-term survival of fat transplants: controlled demonstrations. Aesthetic Plast Surg 1995;19(5):421–5.
8. Coleman SR. Facial recontouring with lipostructure. Clin Plast Surg 1997;24(2):347–67.
9. Allen RJ Jr, Canizares O Jr, Scharf C, et al. Grading lipoaspirate: is there an optimal density for fat grafting? Plast Reconstr Surg 2013;131(1):38–45.
10. Butala P, Hazen A, Szpalski C, et al. Endogenous stem cell therapy enhances fat graft survival. Plast Reconstr Surg 2012;130(2):293–306.
11. Fontdevila J, Guisantes E, Martínez E, et al. Double-blind clinical trial to compare autologous fat grafts versus autologous fat grafts with PDGF: no effect of PDGF. Plast Reconstr Surg 2014;134(2): 219e–30e.
12. Philips BJ, Marra KG, Rubin JP. Adipose stem cell-based soft tissue regeneration. Expert Opin Biol Ther 2012;12(2):155–63.
13. Coleman SR. Structural fat grafting. St. Louis (MO): Quality Medical Pub; 2004.
14. Shaw RB Jr, Kahn DM. Aging of the midface bony elements: a three-dimensional computed tomographic study. Plast Reconstr Surg 2007;119(2):675–81 [discussion: 682–3].
15. Shaw RB Jr, Katzel EB, Koltz PF, et al. Aging of the mandible and its aesthetic implications. Plast Reconstr Surg 2010;125(1):332–42.
16. Shaw RB Jr, Katzel EB, Koltz PF, et al. Aging of the facial skeleton: aesthetic implications and rejuvenation strategies. Plast Reconstr Surg 2011;127(1): 374–83.
17. Coleman SR. Structural fat grafting: more than a permanent filler. Plast Reconstr Surg 2006;118(3 Suppl):108S–20S.
18. Coleman SR. Lower lid deformity secondary to autogenous fat transfer: a cautionary tale. Aesthetic Plast Surg 2008;32(3):415–7.
19. Coleman S. Chin and jawline. In: Coleman S, editor. Structural fat grafting. St. Louis (MO): Quality Medical Pub; 2004. p. 237–92.
20. Coleman S, Saboeiro A, Sengelmann R. A comparison of lipoatrophy and aging: volume deficits in the face. Aesthetic Plast Surg 2009;33(1):14–21.
21. Moratalla Jareno T, González Alonso V, López Blanco E, et al. Use of lipofilling in pediatric patients. Cir Pediatr 2013;26(4):189–94 [in Spanish].
22. Balaji SM. Subdermal fat grafting for Parry-Romberg syndrome. Ann Maxillofac Surg 2014;4(1):55–9.
23. Hunstad JP, Shifrin DA, Kortesis BG. Successful treatment of Parry-Romberg syndrome with autologous fat grafting: 14-year follow-up and review. Ann Plast Surg 2011;67(4):423–5.
24. Coleman SR. Structural fat grafting. Aesthet Surg J 1998;18(5):386, 388.
25. Del Vecchio DA. "SIEF"–simultaneous implant exchange with fat: a new option in revision breast implant surgery. Plast Reconstr Surg 2012;130(6): 1187–96.
26. Del Vecchio DA, Bucky LP. Breast augmentation using preexpansion and autologous fat transplantation: a clinical radiographic study. Plast Reconstr Surg 2011;127(6):2441–50.
27. Kurita M, Matsumoto D, Shigeura T, et al. Influences of centrifugation on cells and tissues in liposuction aspirates: optimized centrifugation for lipotransfer and cell isolation. Plast Reconstr Surg 2008;121(3): 1033–41 [discussion: 1042–3].
28. Eto H, Kato H, Suga H, et al. The fate of adipocytes after nonvascularized fat grafting: evidence of early death and replacement of adipocytes. Plast Reconstr Surg 2012;129(5):1081–92.
29. Khouri RK, Smit JM, Cardoso E, et al. Percutaneous aponeurotomy and lipofilling: a regenerative alternative to flap reconstruction? Plast Reconstr Surg 2013;132(5):1280–90.
30. Orentreich DS, Orentreich N. Subcutaneous incisionless (subcision) surgery for the correction of depressed scars and wrinkles. Dermatol Surg 1995;21(6):543–9.

31. Mojallal A, Lequeux C, Shipkov C, et al. Improvement of skin quality after fat grafting: clinical observation and an animal study. Plast Reconstr Surg 2009;124(3):765–74.

32. Spector JA, Draper L, Aston SJ. Lower lid deformity secondary to autogenous fat transfer: a cautionary tale. Aesthetic Plast Surg 2008;32(3):411–4.

33. Duncan DI, Chubaty R. Clinical safety data and standards of practice for injection lipolysis: a retrospective study. Aesthet Surg J 2006;26(5):575–85.

34. Coleman SR. Avoidance of arterial occlusion from injection of soft tissue fillers. Aesthet Surg J 2002;22(6):555–7.

Primary Breast Augmentation with Fat Grafting

Sydney R. Coleman, MD[a,b,*], Alesia P. Saboeiro, MD[c]

KEYWORDS

- Fat grafting breasts • Breast fat grafting complications • Breast augmentation
- Breast reconstruction

KEY POINTS

- Fat grafting is safe.
- Fat grafting can be used for all types of cosmetic and reconstructive breast procedures, producing soft, natural results.
- Fat is a fragile tissue that must be handled with care to maintain its viability.
- Centrifugation condenses the fat and makes the volumes grafted more predictable and reproducible.
- Fat must be placed into the breast in small aliquots to minimize the chance of fat necrosis.
- Potential complications include fat necrosis and body contour irregularities.
- There is a significant learning curve associated with fat grafting to the breasts.

INTRODUCTION

As early as 1895, Czerny[1] introduced the concept of fat grafting to the breasts when he published an article describing a breast reconstructed using a fist-sized lipoma from the buttock to replace breast tissue removed caused by mastitis. Eugene Holländer[2] began experimenting with fat injections to breasts and in 1912 was the first to describe fat injections to the breast. He showed the correction of not only a missing portion of a breast but also the improvement of scarring of the chest. In 1919, Erich Lexer[3] published his 2-volume book, *Die freien Transplantationen* (translation: free transplantations), which advocated fat grafting for numerous purposes, including correction of breast asymmetry.[3]

After Fournier[4] and Illouz[5] developed the technique of liposuction in the mid-1980s there was renewed interest in fat grafting with the newly acquired semiliquid lipoaspirate. However, in 1987 the American Society of Plastic Surgeons (ASPS) issued a position paper that condemned the practice of fat grafting to the breasts, because they were concerned that the grafted fat would obscure a breast cancer. Sydney Coleman[6–9] began to report his positive experiences with fat grafting to the face and body in the 1990s and emphasized the need for gentle extraction of the fat, purification by centrifugation, and placement of the fat in tiny aliquots to maximize revascularization. He witnessed such reliable results in the male pectoralis muscle, as well as in massive iatrogenic liposuction deformities and buttock augmentation,

Disclosures: Royalties received for instruments sold by Mentor, paid consultant for the Armed Forces Institute of Regenerative Medicine, Mentor Worldwide LLC, and MusculoSkeletal Transplant Foundation (MTF) (S.R. Coleman). No disclosures (A.P. Saboeiro).
[a] Department of Plastic Surgery, New York University Langone Medical Center, New York, NY, USA; [b] Tribeca Plastic Surgery, New York, NY, USA; [c] Private Practice, Tribeca Plastic Surgery, New York, NY, USA
* Corresponding author. New York University Medical Center, NY.
E-mail address: info@lipostructure.com

Clin Plastic Surg 42 (2015) 301–306
http://dx.doi.org/10.1016/j.cps.2015.03.010
0094-1298/15/$ – see front matter © 2015 Elsevier Inc. All rights reserved.

that he decided to perform fat grafting to the breasts in a limited number of patients, and we reported these results in 2007.[10] Our findings showed that breasts can be remarkably enhanced in terms of size and shape with autologous fat. Furthermore, we believed that the grafted breasts could be easily imaged radiologically and that the grafted fat did not hide breast cancer. A few oil cysts and a few calcifications were noted that could be easily distinguished from lesions seen with malignancy. In 2009, Rigotti and colleagues[11] reported no increase in breast cancer recurrence rates in women who underwent breast reconstruction with fat, and more recently it has been reported that radiographic follow-up of breasts grafted with fat is not problematic and should not hinder the procedure.[12–14] With all of this new information on fat grafting to the breasts, the moratorium condemning the procedure has been reversed and the ASPS position statement has been revised.[15] In 2009, the ASPS Fat Graft Task Force stated that, "Fat grafting may be considered for breast augmentation and correction of defects associated with medical conditions and previous breast surgeries; however, results are dependent on technique and surgeon expertise." We think that the Coleman method for fat grafting to the breast is predictable and stable over time, and this is discussed in this article.

TREATMENT GOALS AND PLANNED OUTCOMES

Although optimal breast size is not universal, the usual goal of most breast procedures is to create a breast shape that is pleasing, youthful, and natural. The shape of the female breasts depends on numerous factors, including the underlying rib cage, the pectoralis muscle, the breast parenchyma and subcutaneous fat, and the elasticity of the overlying skin. Not all of these areas can be directly injected with fat, but they can be influenced and disguised with fat. In the breast/chest area, we have used fat grafting in the following clinical presentations:

1. Primary breast augmentation in patients desiring a modest increase of approximately 1 cup size. If the patient has additional body fat and desires more volume, a secondary procedure can be performed (**Figs. 1** and **2**). Placement around existing breast implants is also possible to disguise the edges and improve capsular contractures. In addition, wrinkling and rippling can be disguised with the addition of fat around the implants as well.
2. To take the place of implants that have been removed. There is a size limitation with 1 fat grafting procedure; therefore, a secondary procedure may be necessary (**Fig. 3**). For correction of tuberous breasts and Poland syndrome, the constricted lower pole of the tuberous breast can be preferentially expanded to improve the overall shape, and the missing or atrophic pectoralis muscle and breast in Poland syndrome can be simulated using fat.
3. To provide coverage over a bony sternum or to fill a pectus excavatum.
4. To precisely fill a lumpectomy or biopsy defect.
5. To reverse radiation damage after breast cancer treatment.[11] The apparent stem cell effect of placing fat beneath radiated tissues is healing of the damaged tissue and improving the quality of the skin, often making further reconstruction possible.
6. To reconstruct a breast after mastectomy. If no previous reconstruction has been performed, fat can be used to create the entire breast in multiple stages. If an implant or flap reconstruction has been performed, fat can be placed into specific residual defects.

A

B

C

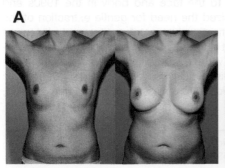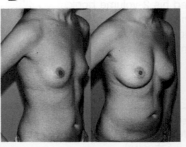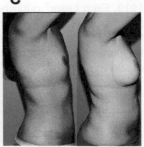

Fig. 1. (*A–C*) A 35-year-old woman who desired larger breasts with a natural feel and slope. She wore the BRAVA device before each of 2 surgeries. She also had a third surgery on 1 breast only. During the first procedure, 232.5 cm³ were placed into the right breast and 230 cm³ were placed into the left. During the second procedure, 272.5 cm³ were placed into the right breast and 287.5 cm³ were placed into the left. During the third procedure, 112.5 cm³ were placed into the lower pole of the left breast only. The total volume placed on the right was 470 cm³, and the total placed on the left was 630 cm³. She is shown before her first surgery and 10 months after the third procedure.

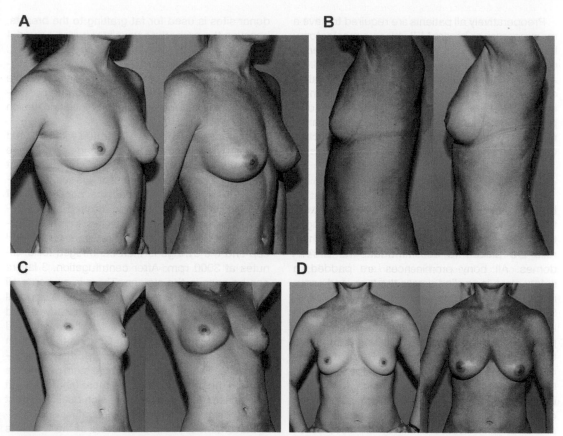

Fig. 2. (*A–D*) A 28-year-old woman who desired larger breasts but was not interested in implants. She wore the BRAVA device before each of 2 surgeries. During the first procedure, 260 cm³ were placed into the right breast and 310 cm³ were placed into the left. During the second procedure, 280 cm³ were placed into the right breast and 270 cm³ were placed into the left. The total volume placed on the right was 540 cm³, and the total placed on the left was 580 cm³. She is shown before the first surgery and 10 months after the second procedure.

PREOPERATIVE PLANNING AND PREPARATION

In many patients, but particularly those who have very small breasts and/or very tight skin envelopes, preoperative and postoperative use of the BRAVA external expansion device seems to significantly improve results.[16] This technique allows the space to which fat can be added to enlarge and, most importantly, increases the blood supply to the existing tissue, making graft take more reliable. The device is worn for 3 to 4 weeks before surgery, including the morning of surgery.

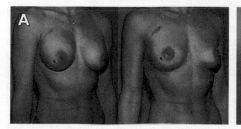
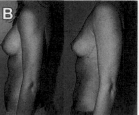
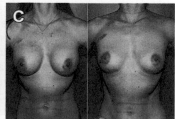

Fig. 3. (*A–C*) A 26-year-old woman who had 300-cm³ saline submuscular implants placed elsewhere 8 years before presenting to our office. She was never happy with the look or the feel of her implants because she thought they were too large for her as well as too high. She desired breasts with a natural feel and appearance. She wore the BRAVA device before her single procedure, during which her implants were removed and replaced with fat. She had 157.5 cm³ placed into the right breast and 142.5 cm³ placed into the left. She is shown before and 8 months after the procedure.

Preoperatively all patients are required to have a mammogram or breast MRI unless a mastectomy has been performed, in which case the patient's oncologist's recommendations are followed. In addition to the mammogram or MRI, preoperative clearance is required, including a history and physical examination, blood work consisting of a complete blood count and prothrombin time/partial thromboplastin time at a minimum, and an electrocardiogram in patients more than 45 years of age.

PATIENT POSITIONING

Patients are brought to the operating room with their BRAVA devices in place. If fat harvesting is to be performed from the prone position, chest rolls are placed to accommodate the BRAVA domes. All bony prominences are padded, a safety strap is applied across the legs, and pneumatic sequential compression booties are applied. Suctioning is performed from the prone position and then the patient is carefully turned into the supine position. If additional suctioning is required, this is completed and then the BRAVA device is removed and the chest is prepped for the placement of the fat. In the supine position, the patient is placed with the hips at the flexion point of the operating table. The patient's arms are extended at 90° on arm boards and they are secured so that the patient can be placed into the sitting position periodically throughout the procedure.

PROCEDURAL APPROACH

All patients wash from the neck down with Hibiclens® soap the night before and on the morning of the surgery. A color-coded system of markings is used to ensure a clear understanding by the patient and the staff as to where the fat will be removed and placed and where the incisions will be made. Green markings are used on the breasts and/or chest to indicate the areas where fat will be placed. Areas to be avoided are marked in orange, such as the midline of the chest or body contour irregularities. Incisions sites are marked in red (~4 mm in length for the placement of fat) and are usually placed in the inframammary crease (1 or 2) and near the nipple or in an existing scar. Fat removal or harvesting is marked in purple and is performed with the goal of enhancing the contours of the body. In very thin women, multiple harvesting sites are often needed in order to obtain enough fat. These incisions are slightly larger (~8 mm) and are placed in natural body creases or stretch marks.

Intravenous sedation with propofol plus the use of local anesthetics and tumescent fluid for the donor sites is used for fat grafting to the breasts, because the procedure usually requires around 4 hours to harvest, process, and reinsert the fat. One dose of intravenous cephalosporin is administered to non–penicillin allergic patients before surgery, but no antibiotics are prescribed postoperatively unless there are signs of infection, which is rare.

The harvesting sites are infiltrated with Lactated Ringer with lidocaine 0.1% and epinephrine 1:400,000. For each 1 cm^3 of anticipated fat removal, approximately 1 cm^3 of this solution is infiltrated. High-powered machine suction is not used. Instead, fat is suctioned by hand using a Coleman harvesting cannula attached to a 10-mL syringe. The cannula is replaced with a Luer-Lok™ cap and the syringe is then centrifuged for 3 minutes at 3000 rpm. After centrifugation, 3 layers can be seen in the syringe. There is an upper oil layer, condensed fat in the center, and a lower local anesthetic/blood layer. The oil is removed and used to lubricate incisions for fat placement, and the lower layer is discarded. Grading the fat then separates the middle fat layer even further, or separating the lowest layer of the most stem cell–dense fat from the upper layer of the more oily, less stem cell–dense fat. In areas where skin quality is most crucial the most stem cell–dense fat is used.

Placement of fat into all levels of the breast is done using a blunt 17-gauge infiltration cannula of either 9 or 15 cm in length. Fat is often placed into the pectoralis major muscle, which provides volume and projection, but it is placement of fat into the more superficial tissues that controls shaping of the breast.

It is essential that fat be placed in very small aliquots to maximize the surface area for revascularization and to minimize the chance of fat necrosis. Approximately 0.25 cm^3 of fat is deposited with each withdrawal of the cannula, which makes the procedure very time consuming. Large boluses of fat greatly increase the chance of fat necrosis, oil cysts, lumps, and calcifications.[17]

Depending on the problem being addressed and the desired final outcome, the volume of fat required can vary significantly. Small depressions in the breast, such as those seen after a biopsy or lumpectomy, may require as little as 25 to 50 cm^3 of fat to improve the contours. However, an average augmentation of 1 cup size requires approximately 250 to 400 cm^3 of fat per breast. After centrifugation of a 10-mL syringe of fat and removal of the oil and local/bloody components, the amount of condensed, usable fat is usually about 4 to 6 cm^3; therefore, twice as much fat than is needed must be suctioned. Because the fat is suctioned by hand, it is time consuming.

All donor and breast incisions are closed with interrupted 4-0 or 5-0 nylon sutures.

POTENTIAL COMPLICATIONS AND THEIR MANAGEMENT

Bleeding and infection are rare, therefore postoperative antibiotics are infrequently prescribed.[18] Potential complications in the breasts include fat necrosis, unacceptable scarring of the incisions, and lack of adequate correction and/or size. Occasionally, fat necrosis presents as a palpable lump, but more often it is seen on mammogram as an oil cyst or calcification. These calcifications can usually be easily distinguished from the speculated pattern of calcifications seen with malignancy. A biopsy is recommended if the findings are indeterminate. If the final breast size or shape is not satisfactory, and the patient has additional fat to be harvested, a secondary fat grafting procedure can be performed once the swelling has resolved; usually in approximately 4 months.

In the donor sites, unacceptable scarring of the incisions can also be an issue. However, by lubricating the incisions using the oil removed from the harvested fat after centrifugation, this can be minimized. Contour deformities in the donor sites are more problematic, but can be corrected using the same fat grafting technique described earlier. Postoperative seromas in donor sites, particularly after suctioning of the so-called love handles or sacrum, can occur and can be managed proactively by leaving the incision (which is usually at the top of the gluteal cleft) open to drainage, or by needle aspiration postoperatively.

POSTPROCEDURAL CARE

Postoperatively, patients are placed into a surgical brassiere and a compression garment is placed on the donor sites. Reston™ foam is occasionally used if the inframammary crease needs stabilization. Cold therapy is not used. Breast and body sutures are removed 5 to 7 days postoperatively and use of the BRAVA device is resumed a few days after surgery if it was used preoperatively. If so, the BRAVA device is worn postoperatively for 2 to 4 weeks.

REHABILITATION AND RECOVERY

Postoperatively, patients generally have moderate bruising, swelling, and discomfort in both the donor sites and the grafted areas; however, this is normal.

The breasts will appear firm and look larger than they will look ultimately. During the first 4 to 6 weeks, most of the swelling resolves; however, small amounts of swelling are likely to remain for up to 4 months.

OUTCOMES

The Coleman technique of fat grafting, which involves hand suctioning of the fat, centrifugation, and meticulous placement, has proved to be consistent and reliable. Preserving the integrity of the fat cells in this manner leads to long-term results. The process is time consuming and labor intensive, making an efficient and well-trained operating staff essential. Faster techniques have been described using suction with higher negative pressures, eliminating the centrifugation phase, and/or injecting fat in significantly larger boluses. However, concerns regarding fat necrosis and inconsistent results with these alternative methods have kept us using the Coleman technique.

CLINICAL RESULTS IN THE LITERATURE

Year	Investigators	Findings
1895	Czerny[1]	1-y stable result after lipoma transfer
1908	Holländer[2]	First injection of fat to the breast
1919	Lexer[3]	Positive results of fat grafting to all areas, including breasts
1995	Coleman and Saboeiro[10]	Positive, predictable results with specific technique

SUMMARY

The acceptance of fat grafting to the breasts by the plastic surgery community has created many possibilities for cosmetic and reconstructive surgeons. Small and large breast defects can be filled; bony prominences and visible implant edges can be disguised; radiation damage can be improved; reconstructions can be refined; difficult breasts can be precisely shaped; implants can be removed and replaced with fat; and a simple, natural augmentation can be performed. It is a time-consuming, meticulous procedure that, although exciting in its range of possibilities, should be done with great care. Novice fat grafting surgeons should start with areas of the face and/or body, such as the hands, that are less complicated or controversial. Only after feeling comfortable grafting fat to other areas should fat grafting to the breasts be attempted; when performed, it should be done in a way that maximizes the potential for graft survival and thus minimizes complications.

REFERENCES

1. Czerny V. Plastischer Erzats de Brustdruse durch ein Lipom. Zentralbl Chir 1895;27:72.
2. Holländer E. Die kosmetische Chirurgie (S.669-712, 45 Abb.). In: Joseph M, editor. Handbuch der kosmetik. Leipzig (Germany): Verlag van Veit; 1912. p. 690–1.
3. Lexer E. Die freien transplantationen. Stuttgart (Germany): Ferdinand Enke; 1919. p. 605.
4. Fournier PF. Reduction syringe liposculpturing. Dermatol Clin 1990;8(3):539–51.
5. Illouz YG. Surgical remodeling of the silhouette by aspiration lipolysis or selective lipectomy. Aesthet Plast Surg 1985;9(1):7–21.
6. Coleman SR. Facial recontouring with lipostructure. Clin Plast Surg 1997;24(2):347–67.
7. Coleman SR. Long-term survival of fat transplants: controlled demonstrations. Aesthet Plast Surg 1995;19(5):421–5.
8. Coleman SR. Lipoinfiltration of the upper lip white roll. Aesthet Surg J 1994;14(4):231–4.
9. Coleman SR. The technique of periorbital lipoinfiltration. Oper Tech Plast Reconstr Surg 1994;1:20–6.
10. Coleman SR, Saboeiro AP. Fat grafting to the breast revisited: safety and efficacy. Plast Reconstr Surg 2007;119(3):775–85 [discussion: 786–7].
11. Rigotti G, Marchi A, Gali M, et al. Clinical treatment of radiotherapy tissue damage by lipoaspirate transplant: a healing process mediated by adipose-derived adult stem cells. Plast Reconstr Surg 2007;119(5):1409–22.
12. Veber M, Tourasse C, Toussoun G, et al. Radiographic findings after breast augmentation by autologous fat transfer. Plast Reconstr Surg 2011;127(3):1289–99.
13. Rigotti G, Marchi A, Stringhini P, et al. Determining the oncological risk of autologous lipoaspirate grafting for post-mastectomy breast reconstruction. Aesthetic Plast Surg 2010;34:475–80.
14. Alvarez S. Natural breast augmentation or fat transfer: the mammographic and sonographic correlation. J Diagn Med Sonogr 2012;28(1):26–32.
15. Gutowski KA, Baker SB, Coleman SR, et al. Current applications and safety of autologous fat grafts: a report of the ASPS Fat Graft Task Force. Plast Reconstr Surg 2009;124:272–80.
16. Del Vecchio DA, Bucky LP. Breast augmentation using preexpansion and autologous fat transplantation: a clinical radiographic study. Plast Reconstr Surg 2011;127(6):2441–50.
17. Eto H, Kato H, Suga H, et al. The fate of adipocytes after nonvascularized fat grafting: evidence of early death and replacement of adipocytes. Plast Reconstr Surg 2012;129(5):1081–92.
18. Coleman SR. Problems, complications and postprocedure care: chapter 4. Structural fat grafting. St Louis (MO): Quality Medical Publishing; 2004. p. 75–102.

Combined Use of Implant and Fat Grafting for Breast Augmentation

Eric Auclair, MD[a], Namrata Anavekar, FRACS[b],*

KEYWORDS

- Composite breast augmentation (CBA) • Retro-fascial pocket • Fat grafting • Shaped implant
- Esthetic breast augmentation

KEY POINTS

- Composite breast augmentation (CBA) offers an attractive alternative to the use of submuscular implants in patients of slender stature.
- CBA has the advantage of providing increased breast volume, while simultaneously maintaining a natural appearance.
- By avoiding submuscular implant positioning, postoperative pain is reduced, as is dynamic movement of the implant.

INTRODUCTION OR OVERVIEW

For over 10 years, numerous investigators have described the successful and extensive use of fat grafting in plastic surgery. The original concept of fat micrografting can be attributed to Coleman. Through his work, liposculpture and its benefits were introduced, initially in the face,[1] followed by grafting to the breast and body.[2] The evolution of micrografting was further supported by the work of Yoshimura and colleagues[3] in their sentinel article discussing cell-assisted lipotransfer for cosmetic breast augmentation. Throughout the history of fat grafting, concerns have been raised regarding its safety in postoperative surveillance of breast architecture. Such concerns have been addressed by Delay and colleagues[4,5] who demonstrated that fat grafting does not in fact interfere with mammographic interpretation. Rubin and colleagues[6] demonstrated that fat grafting of the breast produced fewer radiographic abnormalities and improved Breast Imaging

Reporting and Data System (BI-RADS) scores with less-aggressive follow-up recommendations by breast radiologists when compared with reduction mammoplasty, a widely accepted procedure. Cameron and colleagues[7] had comparable conclusions with their series of patients operated with the CBA technique. The significant contributions of Khouri and colleagues[8] must also be recognized. In this article by Khouri and colleagues,[8] they introduce the BRAVA device (Brava, LLC, a subsidiary of Bio-mecanica Inc, Miami, FL, USA), which, when used in combination with fat grafting, improves fat engraftment by enlarging the capacity of the recipient site and enhancing the vascularity of the breast.

Although this list is by no means exhaustive, it certainly demonstrates the pivotal role fat grafting has in modern plastic surgery and recognizes the numerous surgeons who have contributed to its evolution. Interest in fat transfer is not new, as well summarized by Mazzola elsewhere in this issue. However, it can be said that the first

No disclosures to declare for any authors.
[a] Private Practice, 68 bis Rue Spontini, Paris 75116, France; [b] Clinique Nescens Paris Spontini, 68 bis Rue Spontini, Paris 75116, France
* Corresponding author.
E-mail address: namrata_anavekar@yahoo.com.au

Clin Plastic Surg 42 (2015) 307–314
http://dx.doi.org/10.1016/j.cps.2015.03.005
0094-1298/15/$ – see front matter © 2015 Elsevier Inc. All rights reserved.

plasticsurgery.theclinics.com

technical refinements made by Coleman, followed by many other contributors, have not only significantly improved the quality of results but also broadened the indications.

Simultaneous use of a breast implant and autologous fat grafting is a simple concept, which combines the benefits of effective breast augmentation provided by implants with the remodeling capabilities provided by fat. Even more importantly, this technique obviates retromuscular implant placement in thin patients who present with reduced skin flap thickness. The primary author commenced using this technique in 2006, initially in secondary cases to camouflage visible implants (Case 1; **Fig. 1**), followed soon by use in primary cases (Case 2; **Fig. 2**). Although the author published this technique in 2009,[9] his group further published a series of clinical cases demonstrating the efficacy of this procedure in 2013,[10] thus introducing the term "composite breast augmentation."

TREATMENT GOALS AND PLANNED OUTCOMES

In cases of primary breast augmentation, the aim of CBA is to provide appropriate coverage of the implant in patients who have reduced skin thickness in the presternal area (**Fig. 3**). This coverage then obviates a submuscular pocket and its associated drawbacks (eg, pain and animation with activity). It is desirable to offer patients a single-stage surgery, with minimal downtime. In addition, the final result should appear natural and proportionate.

PREOPERATIVE PLANNING AND PREPARATION
Patient Selection

A thorough history and clinical examination is performed. In particular, a family history of breast cancer precludes the use of fat grafting. The

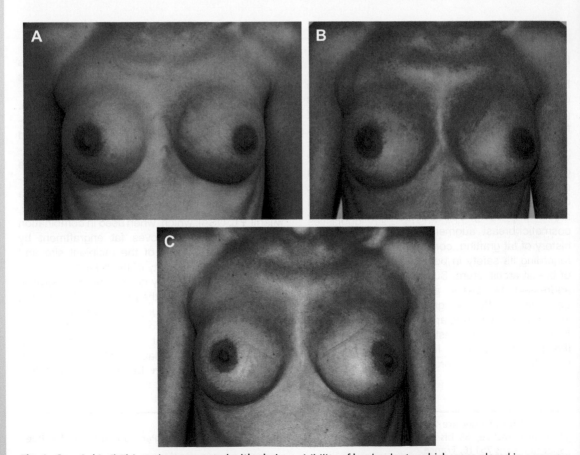

Fig. 1. Case 1: (A–C) This patient presented with obvious visibility of her implants, which were placed in a premuscular plane. She was managed with autologous fat grafting with 80 g to each breast to the areas of visibility. Follow-up at 1 and 5 years demonstrates not only successful camouflage of the implants but also maintenance of the result (A) preoperatively, (B) at 1 year postoperatively, and (C) at 5 years postoperatively.

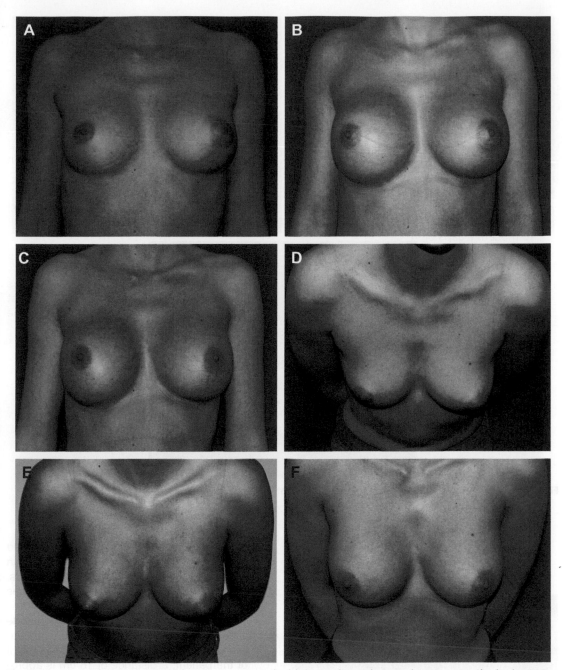

Fig. 2. Case 2: (*A–I*) This 25-year-old patient presented with breast hypoplasia and asymmetry. She had a 270-cc round implant inserted on the right side, with 100 g of autologous fat injected into the anterior aspect of the breast to cover the entire implant. On the left side, she had a 170-cc round implant with no fat grafting required. It can be observed that the symmetry has been stable at 6 months and 1 year postoperatively. (*A–C*) Frontal view preoperatively, at 6 months, and at 1 year. (*D–F*) Patient inclined at 45° preoperatively, at 6 months, and at 1 year.

authors do not use fat grafting in patients older than 40 years with a family history of breast cancer. In addition, the expectations of the patient in terms of volume and shape of the breast must be discussed.

Clinical examination must assess the following:

- Symmetry of the areolas, symmetry and level of inframammary folds (IMFs), and volume of mammary glands.

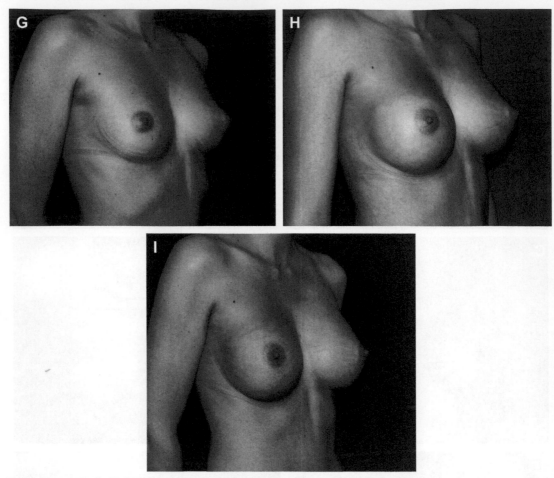

Fig. 2. (continued). (G–I) Oblique lateral view preoperatively, at 6 months, and at 1 year.

- Any rotation of the chest must be noted preoperatively. Failure to do so results in obvious asymmetric projection of the breasts.
- Breast base diameter, which then determines the choice of prosthesis diameter.
- The distance between the nipple and clavicle should be assessed (usually found to be between 14 and 16 cm depending on the height of the patient; a distance of 16 cm is appropriate in a patient 1.75 m tall but would not be suitable in a patient 1.55 m tall).
- The distance between the areola and the IMF helps determine the shape of the implant. To obtain a natural-appearing result, this distance should be greater than 7 cm.

Choice of Implant

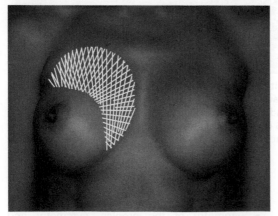

Fig. 3. Fat grafting can be used as a means to camouflage implant visibility, particularly superior and medial to the implant.

One of the advantages of CBA is that it enables the surgeon to sculpt the shape of the breast such that specific anatomic implants are not necessarily required. That is to say, by using round implants one can avoid the complications of implant rotation, yet the anatomic shape can be provided with the addition of fat grafting (**Fig. 4**). In the authors' personal experience, the use of anatomic implants has declined from 50% to less than 10% since the introduction of CBA in his surgical practice. The remaining 10% of patients who still benefit from anatomic implants are those who present with a reduced IMF distance of less than 3 to 4 cms.

In selecting an appropriate implant, the surgeon has increased flexibility if CBA is performed. In contrast, if fat grafting is not used, the dimensions of the implant must be specifically designed to suit the patient, with a limited margin for error.

The two critical measurements in choosing the correct implant are breast diameter and desired breast projection, or, in patient terms, desired cup size. First, regarding breast diameter, the implant width is chosen based on the expected breast width. Second, the achievement of a particular breast cup size can be predicted by knowing that for a given patient who presents with an A cup, an implant projection of 3 cm results in a B cup, a 5-cm implant projection leads to a C cup, and of course a 4-cm projection provides a result in between the two.

PATIENT POSITIONING

Before making a decision regarding patient positioning, one must consider the areas from which fat is to be harvested and whether concomitant liposculpting is to be performed. In the instance where fat is to be harvested either from the buttocks or posterior thighs, the operation must commence with the patient in the ventral position. If, however, sufficient fat can be harvested from the abdomen or the anteromedial thighs, the entire procedure can be performed with the patient in the standard supine position.

Then, in order to facilitate implant insertion, appropriate positioning is vital. The patient's arms should be positioned with 45° of shoulder abduction and 90° of elbow flexion. This position allows efficient

access to the axillary region while not distorting breast position. It should be noted that in certain circumstances (eg, patients with a broad shoulder girdle), the use of armrests might be required.

PROCEDURAL APPROACH
Infiltration

In all of operative regions, infiltration must be provided not only for analgesic requirements but also for liposuction purposes. The components of the infiltration generally include normal saline, a long-acting analgesic, and adrenaline. The specific dosage of these components used in the author's practice is as follows: 400 mL normal saline, mixed with 40 mL of xylocaine 1% with adrenaline, 0.4 mg adrenaline, and 7.5 mg ropivacaine.

Fat Harvesting

A conventional liposuction cannula, 3 to 4 mm in diameter is used to harvest fat. Fat harvesting is performed under low pressure and the material collected via a sterile suction-assisted device. The harvested material is then decanted into several 10-mL syringes, which subsequently undergo centrifugation for 1 minute at 3000 revolutions/minute.

Insertion of Implants

Implant placement is performed via a transaxillary approach. A 4- to 5-cm L-shaped incision is placed at the border of the hair-bearing skin of the axilla. A thick skin flap is raised, and dissection is performed to identify the lateral border of the pectoralis major muscle. Once this has been achieved, the premuscular, retrofascial plane can be entered and the implant pocket can be created, as described by Graf and colleagues[11] and Sampaio Goes.[12] Dissection is done with an illuminated retractor, which enables visualization of the pocket at all times; this ensures adequate control of the dissection, allowing the surgeon to adjust the implant pocket boundaries as required, as well as ensuring optimal hemostasis.

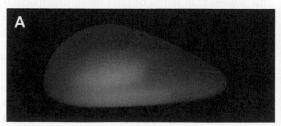
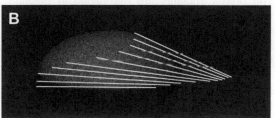

Fig. 4. The image to the right (*B*) demonstrates how the use of fat grafting in combination with a round implant can mimic the shape of an anatomic implant (*A*), whilst maintaining a natural feel to the breast.

Several measures are used to maintain aseptic conditions during implant insertion. First, surgical gloves are changed immediately before implant placement. Furthermore, the implant is handled for a minimum duration. In addition, the implant is bathed in gentamicin.

Once the implant is in a satisfactory position, multilayered wound closure follows. The fascia is closed with a 3/0 monofilament suture, the subcutaneous layer is closed with a 4/0 slow-resorbing suture, and the intradermal layer is closed with a rapidly resorbing 4/0 suture.

Fat Grafting

After implant insertion has been completed, fat grafting can take place with a 16 or 18 gauge, 15 cm long cannula with a single hole just inferior to the tip. The aim of this step is to camouflage the borders of the implant, which may be visible, especially in thin patients. The superior and medial borders of the implant are particularly prone to visibility. Two stab incisions are made: one in the medial aspect of the IMF and the other in the superomedial edge of the areola. Via these incisions, grafting is performed in a radial direction in the subcutaneous plane, being sure to avoid the implant pocket (see **Fig. 3**).

A few technical points should be noted. First, although the majority of patients only require grafting in their cleavage area (ie, superior and medial borders of the implant), a minority of cases warrant grafting to the lateral breast region, as well as in the submammary area in order to prevent a "double bubble" deformity. Also, the volume of fat that is used for grafting is not related to the implant volume - the fat grafts are merely designed to camouflage implant borders, not to increase projection of the breast.

Dressings and Postoperative Management

Dressings not only provide an optimal environment for wound healing but also avoid implant displacement and maximize fat engraftment. The areas, which have undergone fat grafting, are coated with adhesive polyurethane dressing for 1 week. The breast implants are maintained in position with a compressive bandage overnight, which is replaced the following day by a medical bra, which is to be worn continuously throughout the day and night for 3 weeks.

POTENTIAL COMPLICATIONS AND THEIR MANAGEMENT

Complications of this operation are rare and are essentially the same as those for any breast augmentation procedure. Potential postoperative complications are hematoma, implant displacement, and periprosthetic contracture. These complications can be avoided by ensuring adequate hemostasis intraoperatively and by patient compliance with the medical bra. If a hematoma is noted, it must be evacuated early to avoid prolonged blood-implant contact, because this is thought to be a major factor in the development of implant contracture. In addition, the surgical field is completely under vision for the entire procedure, also aiding in hemostatic control.

If implant displacement occurs in the early postoperative period, it may be corrected by external manipulation and use of a compressive bandage for 3 weeks. Periprosthetic contracture may initially be managed with massage. If this fails, surgical management with capsulotomy should be discussed with the patient. Thus far, no cases of wound infection or implant displacement have been reported with this technique.

The incidence of late complications, such as contracture, is similarly low, and this can be attributed to the low hematoma and infection rates observed. Another late complication to consider is fat atrophy. It should be remembered that this cohort of patients is composed of typically thin women with limited excess fat available for harvesting. One must balance the need for fat grafting with the potential for causing unwanted donor site morbidity. Even within these limits, the authors have observed a very low incidence of implant visibility requiring further surgery (2.5% in the authors' series[10]).

POSTPROCEDURAL CARE

It is advised that the patient remain hospitalized overnight, in particular to address any immediate problems, which may arise, such as hematoma. Antibiotics are administered intravenously on induction (2 g cefazolin). No further antibiotic is required. A compressive bandage is applied during this period of hospitalization. On the first postoperative day, this dressing is replaced with a surgical bra, which is to be worn continuously for 3 weeks. In terms of pain relief, oral medications such as paracetamol, as required, provide adequate analgesia.

REHABILITATION AND RECOVERY

Patients are advised to return to work in 2 to 3 days, depending on the conditions of employment. In addition, they are restricted from lifting heavy objects or strenuous sporting activities for 6 weeks. Patients are educated regarding regular massage and shoulder abduction once per day to prevent the development of axillary contracture.

OUTCOMES

Arguably, the most important factor in assessing outcomes is patient satisfaction. Typically, patients are pleased by the enhancement of breast volume, while maintaining a natural feel and appearance, which is provided by the addition of fat grafting. Furthermore, by avoiding any retromuscular dissection, patients rarely complain of pain being a significant issue in their postoperative course.

As other studies have previously noted, 30% of fat transferred undergoes atrophy.[2] The author thus advises to overinject to address this problem. By doing so, one can expect the final result to plateau in its appearance after approximately 6 months. Usually, the donor sites from which fat is harvested do not demonstrate any significant morbidity. On the contrary, patients are pleased with the results of this liposculpture. As discussed previously, the incidence of early and late complications is quite low.

One of the points of contention in fat grafting of the breast is the development of calcifications, which may impact interpretation of mammograms and other radiological imaging. This issue was addressed in a recent publication by Cameron, Auclair and colleagues[7] in which 57 postoperative mammograms after CBA were reviewed by 3 independent radiologists. The findings of this study revealed that no additional imaging or biopsies were required in a 29-month average (range = 0–72 months) follow-up period. In addition, all 52 mammograms were assigned a BI-RADS assessment category 2, indicating benign pathology. This observation demonstrates that autologous fat grafting is in fact a safe technique in esthetic breast surgery, and furthermore, it does not interfere with postoperative interpretation of mammographic imaging.

CLINICAL RESULTS IN THE LITERATURE

At this stage, there are only 2 publications in the medical literature pertaining to composite breast grafting.[9,10] From the article published in 2013 by Auclair and colleagues,[10] the clinical results concerning patients with retrofascial positioning of the implant are summarized in **Tables 1–4**:

In terms of complications, there were 2 cases of capsular contracture. One patient presented 6 months postoperatively and was managed by regular massage of the breasts. The second patient presented 2 years after her original procedure and underwent capsulotomy and further fat

Table 1
Patient demographics

Total number	190
Age (average, range; y)	35 (20–76)
Weight (average, range; kg)	53.7 (45–65)
BMI (average, range)	18.9 (16–22)

Table 2
Implant characteristics

Implant volume (average, range; cc)	270 (150–850)
Round	96
Anatomic	94

Table 3
Details of fat transplantation

Amount harvested (average, range; cc)	550 (150–2000)
Amount injected (average, range; cc)	125 (100–250)
Number of procedures	199

Table 4
Complications

Capsular contracture	2
Additional fat grafting required	9
Hematoma	0
Infection	0

transplantation. This patient has not required any further surgical treatment subsequently.

There were 5 cases in which additional fat grafting was required. All these secondary fat grafting procedures were performed after 6 months. It should be noted, however, that since the publication of this article paper, the first author has performed further revision procedures on an additional 4 cases. These revisions were performed after 1 year (in 3 patients) and 2 years (in 1 patient).

SUMMARY

CBA is a valuable technique in breast esthetic surgery. First, it provides a useful alternative to retromuscular implant positioning in slender patients. By still having the ability to use a premuscular implant pocket, one can avoid the problems of pain, bleeding, implant animation, and bottoming out seen with submuscular breast implants. Furthermore, a premuscular pocket allows more medial positioning of the implant, thus enhancing the visible cleavage. CBA is a safe technique that uses the well-established benefits of autologous fat grafting.

The addition of fat grafting has several advantages. Although implant selection is guided by patient characteristics and expectations, fat transplantation allows optimal results to be achieved by addressing subtle implant visibilities and offering a more natural appearance and feel. Also, central cleavage may be enhanced via the addition of fat in this region. In addition, as many surgeons attest to, it is very difficult to address breast asymmetries solely through the use of implants. It is in such situations that fat grafting proves to be highly useful and effective. This is highlighted in Case 2 (see **Fig. 4**).

CBA is a safe and reliable procedure, with excellent long-term results. These postoperative outcomes are maintained over several years. Patient satisfaction is high, not only with the augmentation result but also with the concomitant liposuction that is required for fat harvesting.

REFERENCES

1. Coleman SR. Facial recontouring with lipostructure. Clin Plast Surg 1997;24(2):347–67.
2. Coleman SR, Saboeiro AP. Fat grafting to the breast revisited: safety and efficacy. Plast Reconstr Surg 2007;119(3):775–85 [discussion: 786–7].
3. Yoshimura K, Sato K, Aoi N, et al. Cell-assisted lipotransfer for cosmetic breast augmentation: supportive use of adipose-derived stem/stromal cells. Aesthetic Plast Surg 2007;32(1):48–55.
4. Delay E, Gosset J, Toussoun G, et al. Delbaere: efficacité du Lipomodelage pour la correction des séquelles du traitement conservateur du cancer du sein. Ann Chir Plast Esthet 2008;53:178–89.
5. Veber M, Tourasse C, Toussoun G, et al. Radiological findings after breast augmentation by autologous fat transfer. Plast Reconstr Surg 2011;127: 1289–99.
6. Rubin J, Coon D, Zuley M, et al. Mammographic changes after fat transfer to the breast compared with changes after breast reduction: a blinded study. Plast Reconstr Surg 2012;129(5):1029–38.
7. Cameron JA, Auclair E, Nelson M, et al. Radiologic evaluation of women following cosmetic breast augmentation with silicone implants and fat grafting. Plast Reconstr Surg 2014;134(4 Suppl 1):91–2.
8. Khouri RK, Eisenmann-Klein M, Cardoso E, et al. Brava and autologous fat transfer is a safe and effective breast augmentation alternative: results of a 6-year, 81-patient, prospective multicenter study. Plast Reconstr Surg 2012;129(5):1173–87.
9. Auclair E. Apport du lipomodelage extraglandulaire dans les augmentations mammaires à visée esthétique (note technique). Ann Chir Plast Esthet 2009; 54:491–5.
10. Auclair E, Blondeel P, Del Vecchio D. Composite breast augmentation: soft tissue planning using implant and fat. Plast Reconstr Surg 2013;132(3): 558–68.
11. Graf RM, Bernades A, Ripple R, et al. Subfascial breast implant: a new procedure. Plast Reconstr Surg 2003;111:904.
12. Sampaio Goes JC, Landecker A. Optimizing outcomes in breast augmentation: seven years of experience with the subfascial plane. Aesthetic Plast Surg 2003;27:178–84.

The Role of Fat Grafting in Breast Reconstruction

Emmanuel Delay, MD, PhD[a,b,*], Samia Guerid, MD[a]

KEYWORDS

- Autologous breast reconstruction • Latissimus dorsi • Lipofilling • Fat grafting • Lipomodeling
- Liposuction • Poland syndrome • Tuberous breast

KEY POINTS

- Careful preoperative clinical and radiologic assessment and clearance for the procedure are mandatory before fat grafting.
- Fat must be transferred in multilayers, starting from the deep plane to the superficial one.
- Fat must be transferred in fine tunnels (like the shape of a spaghetti noodle) in a regular manner to avoid fat necrosis.
- Fat transfer should be interrupted when the recipient site is saturated.
- Resorption rates and fat and recipient site quality must be taken into account to initially overcorrect the volumes.
- Great caution is mandatory when transferring fat in the subclavian region, especially in patients with Poland syndrome, because subclavian vessels may be situated much lower than in normal anatomy.

OVERVIEW

Breast fat transfer is an old concept. In 1895, Czerny described the use of a voluminous lipoma to fill the breast after excision of a fibroadenoma.[1] Several researchers have then used different techniques for breast augmentation and reconstruction.[2–11] The techniques developed at the beginning of the 1980s were controversial. This controversy became so significant after the work of Bircoll,[12–15] and the American Society of Plastic and Reconstructive Surgery released a committee recommendation as follows:

> The committee is unanimous in deploring the use of autologous fat injection in breast augmentation, much of the injected fat will not survive, and the known physiological response to necrosis of this tissue is scaring and calcification. As a result, detection of early breast carcinoma through xerography and mammography will become difficult and the presence of disease may go undiscovered.

This decision was the end of the research and evaluations in this field. Comprehensive debate about this topic can be found in the authors' article published in 2009.[16] Following the work of Coleman[17] depicting the efficacy of fat transfer in the face, we evaluated fat grafting in breast reconstructive and plastic surgery.[18] As the main criticism of fat transfer in breast reconstructive surgery was the potential radiologic consequences, we studied them on a scientific basis.[18] We then applied fat grafting to the different techniques of breast reconstruction, sequelae of conservative breast surgery, and breast malformations.

Disclosures: The authors have nothing to disclose.
[a] Plastic and Reconstructive Surgery Department (University Lyon1), Léon Bérard Center, 28 rue Laennec, 69008 Lyon, France; [b] Private Practice, 50, rue de la République, 69002 Lyon, France
* Corresponding author. Plastic and Reconstructive Surgery Department (University Lyon1), Léon Bérard Center, 28 rue Laennec, 69008 Lyon, France.
E-mail address: emmanuel.delay@lyon.unicancer.fr

Clin Plastic Surg 42 (2015) 315–323
http://dx.doi.org/10.1016/j.cps.2015.03.003

TREATMENT GOALS

Breast and thoracic lipofilling has numerous indications in breast surgery. Breast volume, shape, projection, consistency, and contour can be enhanced with this technique.

Latissimus Dorsi Reconstructed Breasts

Autologous breast reconstruction does not have the implant-related complications and produces a more natural breast. Latissimus dorsi flap transfer without an implant is to us the gold standard technique,[19–21] as it has few postoperative complications and a better molding potential of thoracic volume. In some situations, however, reconstructed volume can be too small. The solution was then to add an implant under the flap. This solution was efficient, but reconstruction was no more autologous. In other situations, global results could be acceptable but some projection was missing or a localized defect prevented the results from being excellent.[22,23] Lipofilling of a reconstructed breast has many advantages: autologous reconstruction process, cost-effectiveness, reproducibility, natural consistency and appearance of the breast, breast symmetry, and last but not least, treatment of fat deposits in the donor regions. Combined with lipomodeling, the autologous latissimus dorsi flap is our first choice in autologous breast reconstruction (**Figs. 1** and **2**).

Latissimus dorsi flap is the most suited fat recipient because of its highly vascularized aspect.[21,22] Our experience showed that a large quantity of fat could be transferred in 1 session (up to 500 mL per breast) with excellent results. Lipofilling is started

from the bone plane to the pectoralis major and then to reconstructed breast, ending in the subcutaneous plane. Patients perfectly understand efficacy and concept of the technique and are then very satisfied with the surgery.

Implant Reconstructed Breasts

Implant reconstructed breast deformities are of 3 types[24]: décolleté asymmetry with step appearance of prosthetic breast, medial deformity with step and too wide intermammary vallée, and lateral deformity with lack of volume above the anterior axillary line. Lipofilling represents 80 to 300 mL. In the décolleté, lipofilling is done in the pectoralis major muscle. In the internal part, lipofilling is in the pectoralis major and between the skin and capsule if implant change is planned. In the lateral aspect, lipofilling can be done only during an implant change, as it is between the skin and capsule (**Fig. 3**).

It seemed to us that fat grafting reduced capsulitis formation, but further studies are needed to prove this effect.

TRAM or DIEP Reconstructed Breasts

Some researchers consider DIEP and TRAM flaps to be excellent breast reconstruction techniques. Some shape and volume defects can, however, be obvious. During the second stage of surgery, intrapectoral and intraflap fat grafting is done, mainly on locations which lack fullness. In some cases, lipofilling is done to increase global flap volume. It is mandatory to transfer less fat in a TRAM or a DIEP than one could do in a latissimus dorsi

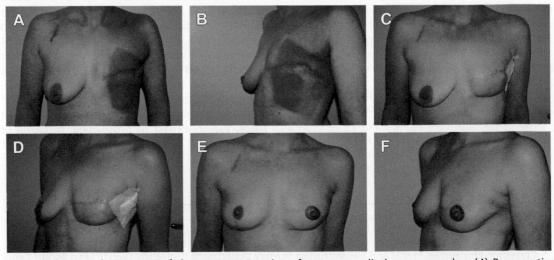

Fig. 1. Patient aged 33 years. Left breast reconstruction after severe radiotherapy sequelae. (*A*) Preoperative view. (*B*) Preoperative oblique view. (*C*) Result immediately after delayed reconstruction with autologous latissimus dorsi flap. (*D*) Postoperative oblique view. (*E*) Final result at 1 year after 1 session of lipomodeling (200 mL) 2 months after the autologous dorsi flap. (*F*) Postoperative oblique view.

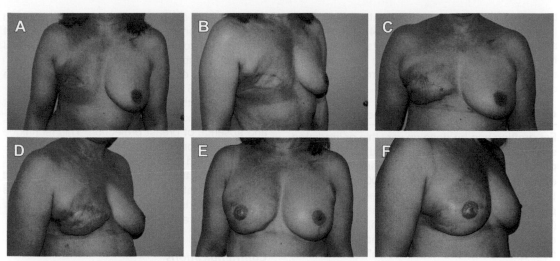

Fig. 2. Patient aged 48 years. Right breast reconstruction. (*A*) Preoperative view. (*B*) Preoperative oblique view. (*C*) Result immediately after delayed autologous latissimus dorsi breast reconstruction. (*D*) Postoperative oblique view. (*E*) Final result at 1 year after 2 sessions of lipomodeling (200 and 400 mL). (*F*) Oblique view.

flap because the former are less vascularized. Another advantage of fat grafting secondary to TRAM or DIEP flap is the possibility to correct abdominal and flanks contour. This also prevent the need of secondary flap mobilization.

Breast Reconstruction with Fat Grafting Only

This technique is best suited for small or medium-sized breasts and patients presenting sufficient fat deposits. In a nonirradiated breast after mastectomy, 3 to 4 sessions are needed to achieve

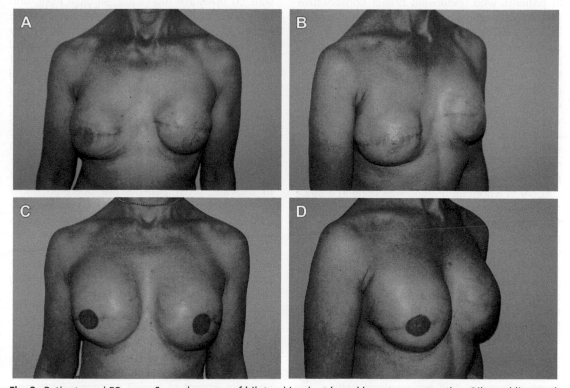

Fig. 3. Patient aged 58 years. Secondary case of bilateral implant-based breast reconstruction. Bilateral lipomodeling (280 mL right, 200 mL left), inframammary fold fixation, and implant changing. (*A*) Preoperative view. (*B*) Preoperative oblique view. (*C*) Postoperative view (1 year). (*D*) Postoperative oblique view.

breast reconstruction with contralateral symmetry. In the presence of radiotherapy, 4 to 6 sessions are needed to obtain optimal results. This protocol has been evaluated[25] and seems interesting for some specific conditions or to correct secondary cases after failed reconstruction.

Other Applications in Breast Reconstruction

Fat grafting can be done on very thin or irradiated skin 2 to 3 months before planned autologous or prosthetic reconstruction to prepare the thoracic area. In this indication, 80 to 200 mL of fat is transferred. Skin quality is enhanced and necrosis prevented. When thoracic malformation is present (eg, lateralized pectus excavatum), lipomodeling can correct deformity and enhance reconstruction and is then a "sur-mesure" (customized) reconstruction. Finally, fat grafting may be done on a native breast to enhance symmetry with a reconstructed breast, mostly in the décolleté region or to slightly increase the volume of the native breast. In this last indication, a preoperative and careful diagnostic imaging is to be done (ultrasonography and mammography) with a control at 1 year.

Corrections of Breast Conservative Surgery

In patients who underwent breast conservative surgery, the technique is done with strict radiologic screening. Risk of coincidence with a new cancer, or a recurrence of the previous one, is high.[26] Our protocol includes an accurate radiologic breast status[27,28] with mammographic, ultrasonographic, and MRI evaluation by an experienced breast imaging specialist. One year postoperatively, we achieve a new radiologic breast status with mammography and ultrasonography. If a suspect lesion is visualized, a microbiopsy is done. One study[27] presented 42 patients with sequellae of breast conservative surgery in whom fat grafting was done in a strict radiologic protocol. The conclusions were that lipomodeling is a huge step in the therapeutic possibilities of surgical management of conservative surgery moderate sequelae.[29] Breast imaging is not affected by the technique, and fat grafting does not prevent an accurate radiologic breast screening. This indication is the most troublesome, and we highly recommend that these patients be treated in a multidisciplinary setting.

Thoracic Malformations

Three indications, in a nononcologic setting, are presented here. Tuberous breasts can be an indication of lipomodeling. This technique can be done alone in about half of cases or in addition to implants or mammaplasty procedures. Fat grafting has, to us, highly modified the surgical treatment of tuberous breasts (**Fig. 4**).[30]

Fat grafting of patients with Poland syndrome is done in 2 to 6 sessions, depending on the importance of the thoracomammary malformation. It corrects the axilla scar, lack of thoracic volume, and absence of breast projection. This technique is, in our opinion, a surgical revolution in the treatment of Poland syndrome.[31,32]

Finally, pectus excavatum is a well-suited indication for fat grafting, and the technique allows one to obtain improvement of thoracomammary shape and excellent breast symmetry.[33]

Contraindications

Contraindications to lipomodeling are unusual.[16] Thin patients with almost no fat deposits can be of concern. Temporary contraindication is fat necrosis in the breast region because the latter is not a suited recipient tissue for fat graft.

PREOPERATIVE PLANNING

Patients are asked to sign a detailed informed consent on operative technique, surgical risks, and potential complications. It is mandatory for the patient to be weight stable at the time of surgery because fat modifies according to the general weight equilibrium. Treated zones on the breast are evaluated and marked on the patient. Natural fat deposits are also evaluated throughout the body and their contours marked on the skin (**Fig. 5**A). Our first choice is abdominal fat because it is appreciated by patients and there is no need to change position during surgery. Our second choices are the saddlebags and internal aspect of thighs and knees. Owing to the quantity of fat to aspirate, most patients are operated under general anesthesia. Often, in breast reconstructive surgery, this step is done at the same time as areolar reconstruction and opposite breast symmetrization. Usual prophylactic antibiotic administration is done perioperatively. Local anesthesia can be given only for small surfaces, mainly during corrections.

PATIENT POSITIONING

Depending on the location of fat deposits, the patient is placed in the prone (hips, buttocks, or posterior aspect of thighs) or supine (abdomen, flanks, anterior aspect of thighs) position. Care is taken to prevent formation of decubitus ulcer.

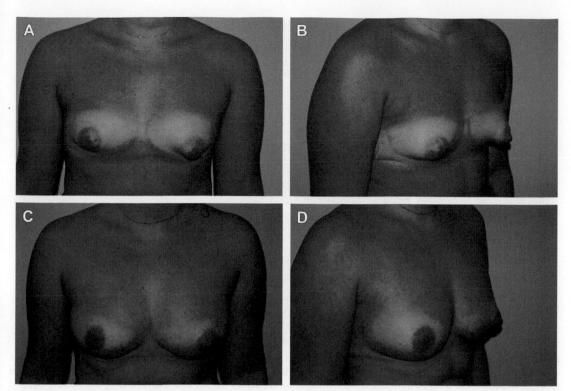

Fig. 4. Patient aged 24 years. Tuberous breast. Correction by 2 sessions of lipomodeling separated by 3 months. Right side, 300 and 300 mL; left side, 350 and 350 mL. (*A*) Preoperative view. (*B*) Preoperative oblique view. (*C*) Postoperative view at 1 year. (*D*) Postoperative oblique view.

PROCEDURAL APPROACH
Incisions

Incisions are made in the skin near the marked fat deposits with a No. 15 blade. The whole area is infiltrated with saline and adrenaline (1 mg adrenaline in 500 mL saline).

Aspiration

Precision at every step of the procedure is important for fat survival in the short, medium, and long term.[2,22] The aspiration cannula has a diameter of 3.5 to 5 mm, with an atraumatic end that can be passed through a 4-mm incision. Aspiration is done using a 10-mL Luer-Lock syringe adapted on the cannula and is done slowly to reduce fat trauma (see **Fig. 5**C). One should be aware that the amount of aspirated fat has to be slightly more than needed to compensate for the loss during centrifugation and months after transfer. Incisions are closed with a thin, fast-resorbable synthetic suture.

Fat Conditioning

After aspiration, surgery staff prepare the syringes for centrifugation: the syringes are capped and centrifuged in a set of 6 (see **Fig. 5**D) for 20 seconds at 3000 rpm.

Centrifugation allows formation of three phases in the syringe (see **Fig. 5**E):

- A top layer containing oil from cellular lysis
- A bottom layer containing blood and infiltration solution
- A central layer, containing purified fat, the useful part of the aspirate

The central layer is transferred, and the others are discarded.

Transfer

Fat transfer is done directly with a 10-mL syringe specifically adapted with a 2-mm-diameter cannula. Multiple incisions, 2 of them in the inframammary fold, are made on the breast with a 18-gauge catheter to cross the transferred fat spaghettis (**Fig. 6**B). Fat grafting is done from a deep to superficial plane to realize a 3-dimensional pattern in the area and prevent the transfer of fat puddle leading to fat necrosis. Transfer is done under low pressure while slowly withdrawing the cannula (see **Fig. 6**C–E). One has to overcorrect the treated area because a 20% to

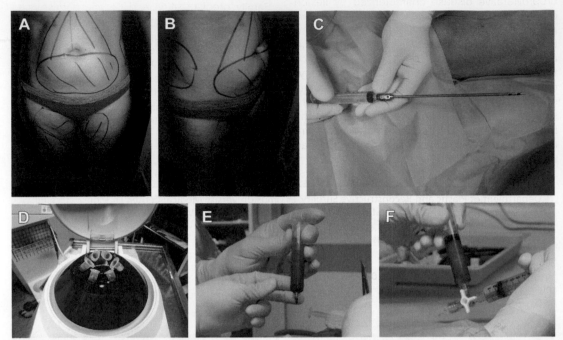

Fig. 5. Fat harvesting and preparation. (*A*) Markings on the donor site. (*B*) Markings on the donor site, oblique view. (*C*) Harvesting with the cannula fitted directly on to the 10-mL Luer Lock syringe. (*D*) Centrifugation of the syringes in batches of 6 for 20 minutes. (*E*) Centrifugation separates the fat into 3 layers. Only the middle layer of purified fat is retained. (*F*) Transfer from one syringe to another, using a 3-way tap to obtain 10-mL syringes containing pure fat.

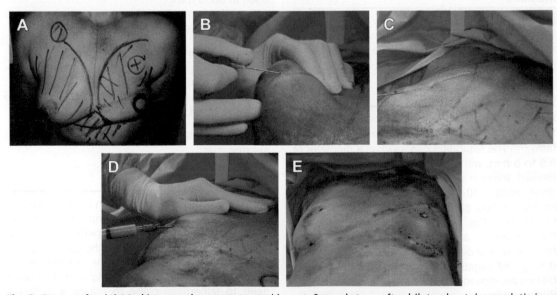

Fig. 6. Fat transfer. (*A*) Markings on the reconstructed breast. Second stage after bilateral autologous latissimus dorsi reconstruction (immediate reconstruction on the right side, delayed reconstruction on the left side). (*B*) Incision in the breast with an 18-gauge trocar. (*C*) Demonstration of the principle of fat transfer: fat is transferred while the cannula is gently withdrawn, leaving a fine cylinder of fat resembling spaghetti. (*D*) Fat transfer into the breast. (*E*) Result at the end of the procedure after 350 mL transfer in the left side and 130 mL transfer in the right side. On the left side, the small incisions left by fasciotomies are seen.

30% fat resorption is to be expected. Once saturation is attained, there is no benefit of further transferring fat, as it leads to fat necrosis. Another session should be planned three months later or more.

COMPLICATIONS AND MANAGEMENT
Aspiration Sites

Incisions have to be placed in a concealed zone, mainly in a skin crease or in the periumbilical area. In the personal series of 2000 cases of the first author (E. D.)and in the 5000 cases of the whole department, we did not have any patient complaining about unaesthetic scars. We had 1 case of flank irregularity needing a secondary correction through lipomodeling of the depression. One local infection has been reported. The clinical presentation was a periumbilical erythema that responded well to antibiotics and local application of cold. There was no aesthetic concern in the final result in the follow-up of those cases.

Breast

Incisions have to be positioned in the inframammary fold or its prolongation in the axilla or in the areolar zone, where scar quality is always excellent. One has to avoid the presternal region, which is more prone to hypertrophy and more noticeable. Because of their small size, scars are almost invisible. In the senior author's (E. D.) 2000 case series, 12 infections have been reported on the breast. The treated zone appeared clinically red, and the corresponding suture was taken out to allow the affected fat to drain. Local care and antibiotics with application of ice allowed complete resolution of infection, with no implication on the final cosmetic result. We had 1 case of intraoperative pneumothorax, probably due to pleura lesion with the cannula. We did not have any case of fat embolization. This complication could happen is fat transfer is done in large vessel, and great caution is mandatory when transferring fat in the subclavian region, especially in patients with Poland syndrome in whom subclavian vessels can be situated at a much lower level than in normal anatomy. We found in 3% of patients a clinically significant fat necrosis and 10% of oil cysts easily treated by puncture at the office. Fat necrosis appears as a firm nodule after lipomodeling. Fat necrosis is clinically very specific: slightly sensitive, stable size, and becoming smaller over time. Increase in the size of a firm breast tumor, even in a reconstructed breast, has to be investigated by a biopsy to rule out malignancy.

POSTPROCEDURAL CARE

Sutures are made with a small-caliber fast-resorbable thread, and a small dry dressing is left in place for a few days.

REHABILITATION AND RECOVERY
Aspiration Sites

Pain at aspiration sites is that of a classical liposuction. Patients complain of severe pain during the first 48 hours, which can be treated with standard oral pain killers. At the end of the aspiration, a solution of ropivacaine is infiltrated, which relieves pain during the first 24 hours. Unpleasant sensitivity can persist for 2 to 3 months. Ecchymosis is significant but disappears in about 3 weeks and postoperative edema in about 3 months.

Breast

Ecchymosis disappears in 15 days and edema in about 1 month. Volume loss is about 20% to 30% of the volume transferred and is stable after 3 to 4 months, subsequently depending on weight stability.

OUTCOMES

Based on the first author's personal experience of 2000 interventions (as of September 15, 2014) and with a 16-year follow-up for the first patients, reliable information on long-term follow-up can be given.

Clinical Long-term Follow-up

All patients were clinically followed up after 15 days, 3 months, and 1 year. Photographs were taken at each consultation. A detailed follow-up protocol to assess objective and subjective quality, patient satisfaction, and any adverse effects or complications was used. The results were considered very good or good in most cases. Few results were considered as moderately good and none as poor. The percentage of good or very good results depends on the subpopulation studied in relation to the indication. For example, for correction by lipomodeling of sequellae of conservative treatment, there were 50% very good, 40% good, and 10% moderately good results.[26]

Patients who had had breast cancer and underwent lipomodeling after conservative treatment or breast reconstruction were then followed up by their oncologist, who referred them to us if there was any change. For the other patients, quality long-term follow-up was made possible by shared computerized medical records.

Radiologic Long-term Follow-up

In 1998, when we developed this protocol, the main fear concerning fat transfer in the breast was the risk that it would compromise imaging investigations. This fear had in fact led to the controversy of 1987 and its consequences, mentioned in the introduction. For this reason, we analyzed the effect of fat transfer on breast imaging. We carried out 3 studies: imaging of breasts reconstructed by autologous latissimus dorsi flap and lipomodeling (mammography, ultrasonography, MRI),[18] imaging of conserved breasts after lipomodeling (mammography, ultrasonography, MRI),[34] and imaging of native breasts with defects corrected by lipomodeling (asymmetry, tuberous breasts, Poland syndrome).[28]

Our findings showed that if lipomodeling was carried out in accordance with modern principles of fat transfer, it in no way hindered breast imaging. We are speaking here of a surgical team that has completed its learning curve and of specialized radiologists who are familiar with the images potentially induced by fat transfer. These results are of fundamental importance to allow the use of fat transfer in aesthetic surgery in native breasts.

Imaging results in most reconstructed breasts were normal, with some images of oily cysts and fat necrosis. All the images observed were in favor of benign lesions easily distinguished from suspicious lesions. Abnormal images were essentially oily cysts, occurring in 15% of cases. The most complex situation concerned lipomodeling for the sequelae of conservative treatment, as in this population fat necrosis already develops in about 20% of patients following the conservative treatment and lipomodeling doubles this rate by generating mainly oily cysts but sometimes more complex lesions of fat necrosis. The experience helps to transfer correct volume of fat depending the quality of the tissues. Because of the spontaneous local recurrence rate of 1.5% per year, surveillance must be rigorous. We believe that this indication should be restricted to multidisciplinary teams working with radiologists who have perfect mastery of the subject.

Oncologic Long-term Follow-up

Sixteen years of oncologic follow-up have not revealed an increased risk of local recurrence after mastectomy or after conservative treatment. Lipomodeling even seems to lower recurrence rate. But to confirm this clinical impression, more complex oncologic studies must be performed that match treated populations with reference populations with the same oncologic status.

SUMMARY

Breast lipomodeling, or breast fat transfer, is a huge step in reconstructive surgery and represents, in our opinion, one of the most important steps of the last 20 years. In autologous breast reconstruction, lipomodeling is the ideal complement of autologous latissimus dorsi flap, allowing breast reconstruction to be completely autologous. Breast lipomodeling can also be used during implant-based breast reconstruction or after TRAM or DIEP flap. Being a huge step in therapeutic choices in treating moderate sequelae of breast conservative surgery, this technique is, in our point of view, only to be used in a multidisciplinary setting to limit potential medicolegal bias in case of outbreak of new cancer occurrence. Finally, breast lipomodeling is prone to greatly change results and indications of thoracic malformations, such as tuberous breasts, breast asymmetry, pectus excavatum, and Poland syndrome.

REFERENCES

1. Czerny V. Plastischer ersatz der brustdrüse durch ein lipom. Zentralbl Chir 1895;27:72.
2. Sinna R, Delay E, Garson S, et al. La greffe de tissu adipeux: mythe ou réalité scientifique. Lecture critique de la littérature. Ann Chir Plast Esthét 2006;51:223–30.
3. Illouz YG. The fat cell "graft": a new technique to fill depressions. Plast Reconstr Surg 1986;78:122–3.
4. Bames HO. Augmentation mammaplasty by lipotransplant. Plast Reconstr Surg 1953;11:404–12.
5. Longacre JJ. Use of local pedicle flaps for reconstruction of breast after subtotal or total extirpation of mammary gland and for correction of distortion and atrophy of the breast due to excessive scar. Plast Reconstr Surg 1953;11:380–403.
6. Illouz YG. La sculpture chirurgicale par lipoplastie. Paris: Arnette; 1988. p. 407.
7. Fournier PF. The breast fill. In: Fournier PF, editor. Liposculpture: the syringe technique. Paris: Arnette Blackwell; 1991. p. 357–67.
8. Schorcher F. Fettgewebsverpflanzung bei zu kleiner Brust. Munch Med Wochensch 1957;99:489.
9. Hang-Fu L, Marmolya G, Feiglin DH. Liposuction fatfilant implant for breast augmentation and reconstruction. Aesthetic Plast Surg 1995;19:427–37.
10. Pohl P, Uebel CO. Complication with homologous fat grafts in breast augmentation surgery. Aesthetic Plast Surg 1985;9:87.

11. Rosen PB, Hugo NE. Augmentation mammaplasty by cadaver fat allografts. Plast Reconstr Surg 1988;82:525–6.

12. Bircoll M. Cosmetic breast augmentation utilizing autologous fat and liposuction techniques. Plast Reconstr Surg 1987;79:267–71.

13. Bircoll M, Novack BH. Autologous fat transplantation employing liposuction techniques. Ann Plast Surg 1987;18:327–9.

14. Bircoll M. Autologous fat transplantation. Plast Reconstr Surg 1987;79:492–3.

15. Bircoll M. Autologous fat transplantation to the breast. Plast Reconstr Surg 1988;82:361–2.

16. Delay E, Garson S, Toussoun G, et al. Fat injection to the breast: technique, results, and indications based on 880 procedures over 10 years. Aesthet Surg J 2009;29:360–76.

17. Coleman SR. Facial recontouring with lipostructure. Clin Plast Surg 1997;24:347–67.

18. Pierrefeu-lagrange AC, Delay E, Guerin N, et al. Evaluation radiologique des seins reconstruits ayant bénéficiés d'un lipomodelage. Ann Chir Plast Esthét 2006;51:18–28.

19. Delay E, Gounot N, Bouillot A, et al. Reconstruction mammaire par lambeau de grand dorsal sans prothèse. Expérience préliminaire à propos de 60 reconstructions. Ann Chir Plast Esthét 1997;42: 118–30.

20. Delay E, Gounot N, Bouillot A, et al. Autologous latissimus breast reconstruction. A 3-year clinical experience with 100 patients. Plast Reconstr Surg 1998; 102:1461–78.

21. Delay E. Breast reconstruction with an autologous latissimus flap with and without immediate nipple reconstruction. In: Spear SE, editor. Surgery of the breast: principes and art. 2nd edition. Philadelphia: Lippincott Williams and Wilkins; 2006. p. 631–55.

22. Delay E. Lipomodeling of the reconstructed breast. In: Spear SE, editor. Surgery of the breast: principes and art. 2nd edition. Philadelphia: Lippincott Williams and Wilkins; 2006. p. 930–46.

23. Delay E. Breast deformities. In: Coleman SR, Mazzola RF, editors. Fat injection: from filling to regeneration. Saint Louis (MO): Quality Medical Publishing (QMP); 2009. p. 545–86.

24. Delay E, Delpierre J, Sinna R, et al. Comment améliorer les reconstructions par prothèses? Ann Chir Plast Esthét 2005;50:582–94.

25. Delaporte T, Delay E, Toussoun G, et al. Reconstruction mammaire par transfert graisseux exclusif. A propos de 15 cas consécutifs. Ann Chir Plast Esthét 2009;54:303–16.

26. Delay E, Gosset J, Toussoun G, et al. Efficacité du lipomodelage pour la correction des séquelles du traitement conservateur du cancer du sein. Ann Chir Plast Esthét 2008;53:153–68.

27. Gosset J, Guerin N, Toussoun G, et al. Aspects radiologiques des seins traités par lipomodelage après séquelles du traitement conservateur du cancer du sein. Ann Chir Plast Esthét 2008;53:178–89.

28. Veber M, Tourasse C, Toussoun G, et al. Radiological findings after breast augmentation by autologous fat transfer. Plast Reconstr Surg 2011;127: 1289–99.

29. Delay E. Correction of partial breast deformities with the lipomodeling technique. Chapter 78. In: Kuerer H, editor. Kuerer's breast surgical oncology. New York: Mac Graw-Hill; 2010. p. 815–25.

30. Delay E, Sinna R, Ho Quoc C. Tuberous breast improvement with fat grafting. Aesthet Surg J 2013;33:522–8.

31. Delay E, Sinna R, Chekaroua K, et al. Lipomodeling of Poland's syndrome: a new treatment of the thoracic deformity. Aesthetic Plast Surg 2010;34: 218–25.

32. La Marca S, Delay E, Toussoun G, et al. Correction de la déformation thoraco mammairee du syndrome de Poland par la technique de lipomodelage : à propos de 10 cas. Ann Chir Plast Esthét 2013;58:60–8.

33. Ho Quoc C, Delaporte T, Meruta A, et al. Breast asymmetry and pectus excavatum improvement with fat grafting. Aesthet Surg J 2013;33:822–9.

34. Gosset J, Flageul G, Toussoun G, et al. Lipomodelage et correction des séquelles du traitement conservateur du cancer du sein. Aspects médico-légaux. Le point de vue de l'expert à partir de 5 cas cliniques délicats. Ann Chir Plast Esthét 2008;53: 190–8.

Tissue-Engineered Autologous Breast Regeneration with Brava®-Assisted Fat Grafting

CrossMark

Tomasz R. Kosowski, MD[a,*], Gino Rigotti, MD[b],
Roger K. Khouri, MD[a]

KEYWORDS

- Tissue engineering • Tissue expansion • Biological scaffold • Brava • Brava + AFT
- Breast reconstruction • Autologous fat transfer • Fat grafting

KEY POINTS

- For large volumes of fat graft to survive, it is necessary to prepare a well-vascularized, large-volume recipient site.
- External tissue expansion with Brava can generate an in situ biological scaffold that will accept a large volume of fat graft required for breast reconstruction.
- With the Brava-assisted technique, it takes an average of 2.8 grafting procedures to regenerate a nonradiated breast mound, while radiated defects require an additional 2.1 procedures to reverse the radiation damage.
- Brava + autologous fat transfer is a minimally invasive, incisionless, safe, economic, attractive, and effective alternative method of breast reconstruction.

INTRODUCTION

Nearly 300,000 American women are diagnosed with breast cancer every year,[1] with 118,000 opting for breast reconstruction after mastectomy. Most reconstructions are implant-based (69%), whereas the remainder are autologous flap reconstructions (31%). Over the past 7 years, the authors have offered a third alternative to more than 400 women who wished to avoid prosthetic material and invasive flap surgery.[2]

The authors' experience has shown that Brava-assisted external tissue expansion with subsequent autologous fat transfer (AFT) is a safe and effective minimally invasive method of regenerating a breast mound.[3] The procedure has the added benefits of restoring a sensate breast mound with minimal morbidity and of body contour improvement through liposuction.

Brava® (Coconut Grove, FL, USA), a well-established vacuum-based external breast expander, applies a distractive mechanical force that induces the body to generate its own 3-dimensional (3D) vascularized scaffold.[3–10] It not only expands the skin defect to generate the necessary skin envelope, but it also stimulates the growth of native stromal and vascular elements. Appropriate expansion creates a larger and more favorable recipient site where many more microdroplets of fat can be diffusely injected without coalescence and without significantly increasing interstitial fluid pressure (**Fig. 1**).[11,12]

The authors' published experience with Brava + AFT for primary breast augmentation and large volume fat transfer established the attractiveness, safety, and efficacy of this technique.[6,13] The authors hereby review their outcomes for Brava + AFT breast reconstruction in 3 patient population

---

[a] Miami Breast Center, Key Biscayne, FL, USA; [b] Clinica San Clemente, Mantava, Italy
* Corresponding author.
E-mail address: tkosowski@gmail.com

Clin Plastic Surg 42 (2015) 325–337
http://dx.doi.org/10.1016/j.cps.2015.03.001
0094-1298/15/$ – see front matter © 2015 Elsevier Inc. All rights reserved.

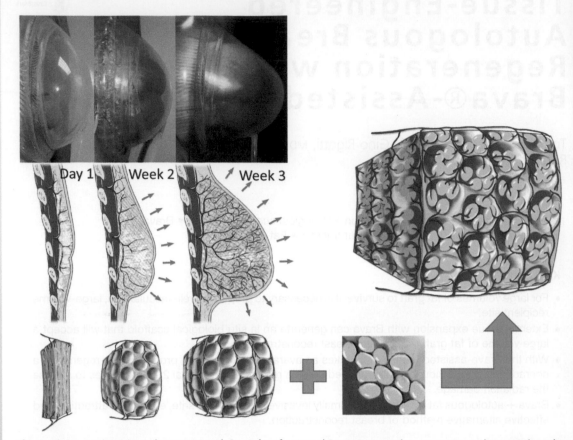

Fig. 1. Tissue engineering a breast mound: 3 weeks of external Brava® expansion generates a tissue engineering scaffold with a rich capillary vascular network that can be seeded with fat microdroplets to generate a well vascularized fatty breast mound.

subsets: delayed reconstruction, immediate reconstruction, and reconstruction of the radiated partial mastectomy defect. Each subset has unique characteristics that must be considered when undergoing Brava + AFT reconstruction.

DELAYED RECONSTRUCTION

In the delayed reconstruction, the patient undergoes 2 to 3 weeks of Brava-mediated tissue expansion in preparation for fat transfer. Tight mastectomy defects limit the amount of fat that can be safely grafted per session, more so in noncompliant, irradiated skin. Brava helps mitigate these effects, thereby decreasing the necessary number of grafting sessions required to complete the reconstruction.[13] **Fig. 2** demonstrates a case of delayed reconstruction.

IMMEDIATE RECONSTRUCTION

Although initially lacking the benefits of expansion, immediate breast reconstruction confers 3 main

advantages[11]: (1) because the recipient muscle is exposed, fine graft ribbons can be carefully teased in between the muscle fascicles under direct vision, which is a huge advantage compared with traditional fat grafting where the surgeon cannot see graft coming out of the cannula; (2) with the investing fascia that normally restricts muscle expansion removed as part of the mastectomy, the recipient muscle can accept a large amount of graft and significantly swell without increasing its interstitial tissue pressure; and (3) closure of the wound allows the plastic surgeon to tailor the amount of residual skin deemed necessary for the optimal reconstruction. Although counterintuitive, excess skin leads to problematic folds that are difficult to subsequently release. Usually 100 to 400 mL of fat can be grafted in the submuscular and intramuscular planes and, if feasible, the base of the mastectomy flaps. With most of the grafts deposited in the upper pole, the patient wakes up with a moderate-sized medial breast mound. This "social breast" helps reduce some of the psychological trauma of the mastectomy. Four to

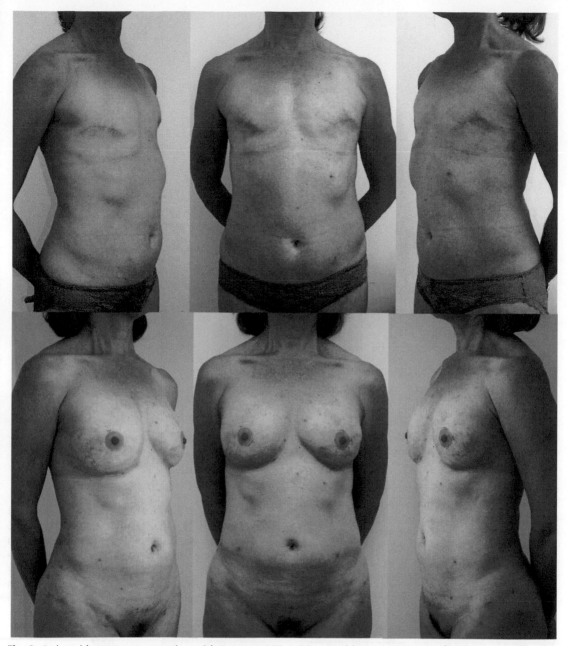

Fig. 2. Delayed breast reconstruction with Brava + AFT. A 52-year-old woman presents for reconstruction after mastectomy for right-sided breast cancer with contralateral prophylactic mastectomy (*top row*). Three sessions of Brava expansion with fat grafting were required to regenerate her breast mounds. Follow-up at 1 year after her final procedure is shown (*bottom row*).

6 weeks after the mastectomy, once the skin flaps have healed and adhered to the grafted muscle, the patients start Brava expansion to further expand the recipient scaffold in preparation for the 1 to 6 additional grafting procedures that might be required to complete the reconstruction. If radiation was planned after mastectomy, immediate reconstruction is not offered because radiation

would damage the grafted fat. **Figs. 3–7** show examples of immediate reconstruction.

RECONSTRUCTION OF LUMPECTOMY DEFECTS

In the radiated lumpectomy, AFT immediately after completing radiation seems to have a soothing

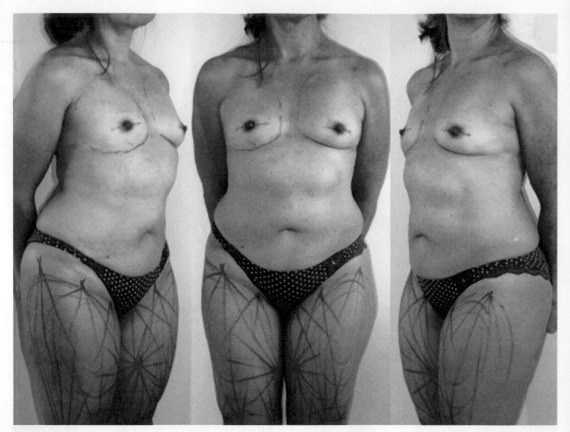

Fig. 3. Preoperative photos of 48-year-old woman before her planned bilateral mastectomy for right breast carcinoma and immediate breast reconstruction with fat grafting.

effect on the radiation-induced inflammation, and the interposed healthy grafts reduce the amount of secondary fibrosis, causing the radiated tissues to remain softer.[14] In addition to serving as a volume filler, fat reduces fibrosis and has a regenerative effect on skin,[15] nerves,[16] and blood vessels.[17] **Figs. 8–10** show examples of reconstruction of lumpectomy.

PATIENT SELECTION AND PREPARATION

Patients have to tolerate a 20-minute in-office test trial of Brava use, understand its use and benefits, and comply with its wear schedule. Exclusion criteria include smoking, prolonged bleeding, multiple previous liposuctions, and unrealistic expectations. Because the authors can harvest a thin

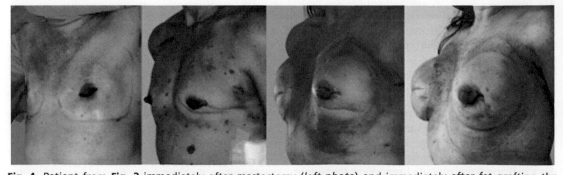

Fig. 4. Patient from **Fig. 3** immediately after mastectomy (*left photo*) and immediately after fat grafting the exposed pectoralis muscle and mastectomy skin flaps (*second from left*). Following additional resection of her right nipple areola complex for a positive margin, Brava expansion of the mastectomy before second (*second from right*) and third (*right*) reconstructive procedures.

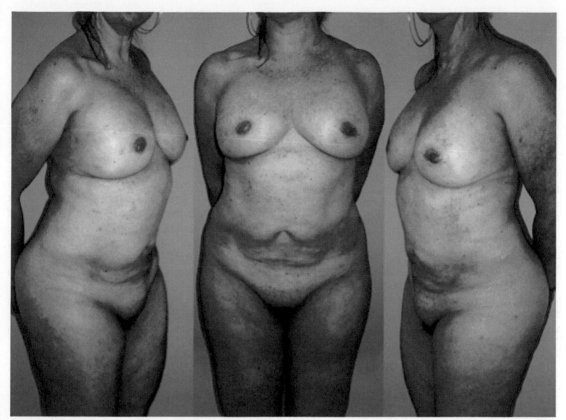

Fig. 5. One-year postoperative result. In addition to appearance to regenerated breast mounds, note the contour improvement of the thigh and flanks donor areas.

layer of fat out of a large expanse, patients with low body mass index (BMI) have excellent outcome and are rarely turned down. Because prior radiation or scarring from previous failed procedures requires significantly more time and expertise, the best candidates for the beginner surgeon are unscarred, unradiated mastectomy defects in patients with moderate fat depots. Patients are required to wear Brava with 60- to 0-mm Hg cycling pressures (3 minutes on/1 minute

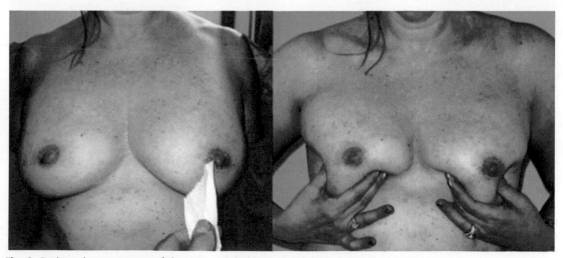

Fig. 6. Patient demonstrates soft breasts with light touch sensation over the nipples.

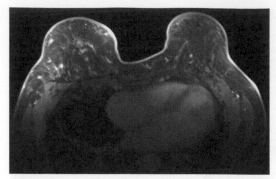

Fig. 7. After reconstruction, MRI of patient shows well-vascularized normal-appearing fat with only a solitary, subcentimeter oil cyst in left breast.

off) for at least 10 hours a day 2 to 3 weeks before their scheduled surgery and are considered well prepared for grafting if the mastectomy defect volume immediately after Brava removal is more than or equal to 2.5 times the pre-expansion volume.

SURGICAL TECHNIQUE

The authors' AFT technique with the Lipografter® (Lipocosm, LLC, Key Biscayne, FL, USA) has previously been described.[13] Briefly, fat is manually liposuctioned using a 12-hole, 12-G cannula connected to the K-VAC® spring-loaded syringe, which provides a 300-mm Hg constant vacuum. Harvesting is efficient because there is no need to switch syringes; recocking the K-VAC® syringe plunger spring automatically sends the lipoaspirate to a collection bag through a 2-way atraumatic tissue valve (AT-Valve®). Once filled, the bag containing the lipoaspirate is centrifuged at 15 G for 1 to 2 minutes (or allowed to sediment at 1 G for 15 minutes). There is very little, if any, free oil with this gentle handling. After draining the infranatant fluid, the supernatant fat is concentrated in the same bag, ready for reinjection (**Fig. 11**).

The authors diffusely reinject the graft through multiple hypodermic needle puncture entry sites using a 14-G single-hole spatulated tip curved

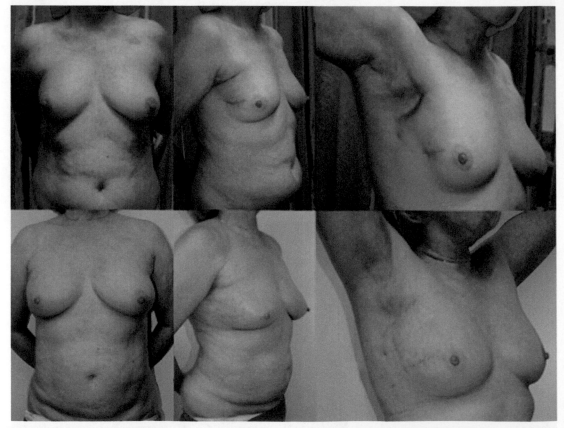

Fig. 8. Preoperative (*top row*) to postoperative (*bottom row*) appearance of a 45-year-old woman with right-sided radiated lumpectomy. She required 2 Brava + AFT procedures. Note the improved and lengthened lateral mammary scar, the medialization of the nipple-areola complex, and the correction of her axillary hollow. Most striking to this patient, however, is the total resolution of her severe antecostobrachial nerve neuritis.

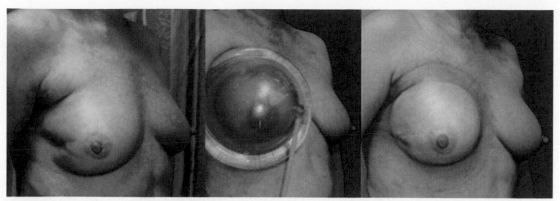

Fig. 9. Lateral view of the right radiated lumpectomy defect: Left, pretreatment; center, with the Brava placed horizontally to recruit more of the lateral breast; right, following 3 weeks of Brava expansion and immediately after removing the device. Brava loosened out the scar contracture, improved the contour defect, and increased the recipient size and its mechanical compliance, and the visible hyperemia reflects an overall increased vascularity of the recipient.

cannula. With a 3-mL syringe, the authors deliver about 0.1 mL/cm through 10- to 30-cm passes of the grafting cannula, injecting as they retract and fanning the mastectomy defect with contiguous arcuate sweeping passes in multiple planes through multiple entry sites. The goal is to diffusely deliver the graft as a fine mist of individual 2-mm droplets through multiple sprinklers to avoid coalescence of the droplets into lakes too wide to revascularize. The AT-Valve® connected to the syringe automatically redraws lipoaspirate from the bag, avoiding the wasted motion of multiple syringe switching. This closed system adheres to accepted principles of fat grafting while saving time and resources.[18] It is important to avoid "overgrafting," which increases interstitial pressure to levels that restrict capillary perfusion (>9 mm Hg).[19,20]

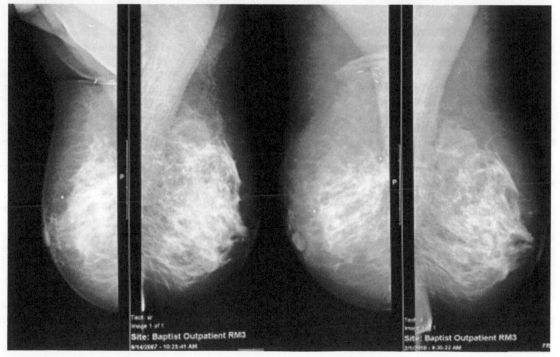

Fig. 10. Preoperative (*left*) and postoperative (*right*) mammogram of patient. Note correction of the axillary cleft and the improved radiolucency of breast.

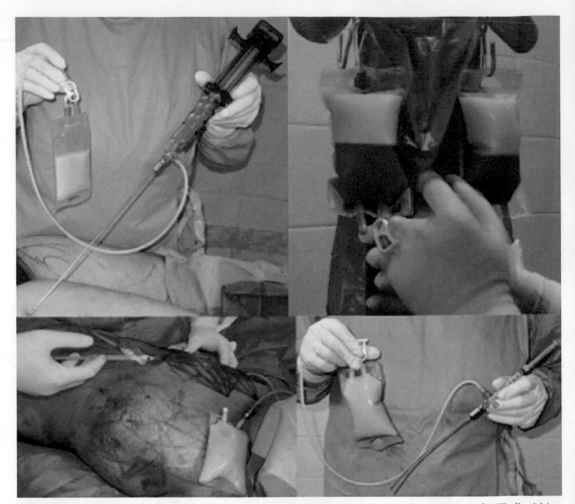

Fig. 11. The Lipografter® device allows for atraumatic harvest, preparation, and reinjection of AFT all within a closed system. (*left upper corner*) In the harvesting mode, the Lipografter consists of a 12-gauge, 12-hole harvesting cannula connected to the K-VAC® spring-loaded syringe through the AT-Valve®. The liposuctioned fat is drawn into the K-VAC® syringe as its plunger is automatically pulled up by the ribbon springs at a constant 300-mm Hg vacuum pressure. Pushing the plunger back down recocks the springs as the AT-Valve® automatically sends the lipoaspirate to the collection bag. (*right upper corner*) Once full, the collection bag is hung on an intravenous pole covered by a sterile drape with hangers made out of folded sterile endotracheal stylets. After sedimenting for about 10 minutes, the fluid is drained and the supernatant fat is concentrated in what becomes the reinjection bag. This gentle harvesting and preparation method produces little to no free oil. (*right lower corner*) In the grafting mode, the Lipografter has a gently curved 14-G, single-hole, spatulated tip grafting cannula connected to a 3-mL syringe by means of the AT-Valve® switched to the grafting mode such that AFT automatically flows from bag to syringe to patient in the direction of the arrows. (*left lower corner*) Breast reconstruction now consists of reinjecting AFT into the expanded mastectomy scaffold. Through multiple 14-G needle puncture entry sites, the authors reinject about 2 mL per 20-cm pass leaving behind 0.1 mL/cm arcuate contiguous ribbons of fat in multiple planes. Thanks to the valve, the AFT can be repeatedly aspirated from the reinjection bag into a fine syringe and automatically reinjected back through the cannula in tiny precise packages while eliminating the time wasted switching cannulas and refilling syringes.

On the third to fourth postoperative day, the patient resumes the constant low-pressure (20 mm Hg) of the Brava Smartbox® for as many hours per day as practically tolerated for 3 to 4 weeks. This acts as a 3D stent to immobilize the grafts and hold the breasts in the expanded state. For

bilateral reconstruction, successful completion is defined as the point at which both the surgeon and the patient are satisfied with the results. For unilateral reconstruction, successful completion is defined as the point at which the size and contour of the reconstructed breast closely matches the contralateral side. If the patient was still not satisfied with the reconstruction at 2 months postoperatively, she resumes Brava expansion for 2 to 4 weeks at the higher cycling pressures to further expand the breast and prepare it for the next AFT (see **Figs. 4** and **9**). The minimum time between procedures is 8 weeks. For an irradiated breast, the minimum time is 3 months.

The authors often use the percutaneous aponeurotomy and lipofilling (PALF) procedure[21] to release surgical scars and the reverse abdominoplasty and fat transfer technique to recruit abdominal tissue and define the mammary folds.[22]

DATA COLLECTION AND ANALYSIS

Demographic data, operative data (volume of grafted fat, number of procedures), perioperative complications as well as breast cancer recurrence were tracked. Breast volumes were determined by 3D imaging.[23] All lumpectomy patients had a baseline and 6-month follow-up MRI. Mastectomy patients had postoperative MRIs taken to work up palpable noncystic masses.

Medicare national average reimbursement data were used in the authors' cost analysis of Brava + AFT, DIEP/TRAM flaps, and tissue-expander/implant-based breast reconstruction.[24–31]

CLINICAL EXPERIENCE

The authors' patient population had a mean BMI of 23.5 (range 15–34) with an average age at first surgery of 28 to 74 years (mean, 45). Mean follow-up was 2.5 years (range, 6 months to 7 years). Of the 488 patients enrolled (1877 AFTs on 616 breasts), 427 patients (87.5%) completed reconstruction (1790 operations on 568 breasts). Of 397 breasts undergoing delayed reconstruction, 71 had at least one previously failed reconstruction with

implants or flaps. Of the 80 breasts that completed immediate reconstruction, 27 were prophylactic.

Delayed nonradiated mastectomies required 2.8 (range, 2–6) procedures to complete reconstruction, whereas delayed radiated mastectomies required 4.9 (range, 3–10) procedures. Prior flap or implant reconstruction failures had more scar tissue and account for the higher range of procedures. Immediate reconstruction required 2.1 grafting sessions (range, 1–5) when nonradiated and 4.2 grafting sessions (range, 2–7) when the breast was previously irradiated. Reconstruction of the radiated lumpectomy defects required 2.0 grafting sessions (range, 1–4). Mean volume of grafted fat was 225 mL per breast per operation. At the initial sessions, although the recipient sites were smaller and stiffer, the authors grafted less than in subsequent sessions when the sites became larger and more compliant. Final mean breast mound volume achieved was 375 mL per breast.

Light touch sensation (detected with a cotton wisp) over the entire surface of the regenerated breast mound was restored in all immediate reconstructions and nonradiated reconstructions with no previous failed reconstruction attempts (see **Fig. 6**). Patient satisfaction with the volume, contour, and feel of their breasts was high at 97%. Barring complications, all patients returned to a desk job activity level after their first postoperative visit (4–5 days).

Complications are presented in **Table 1** and included 5 pneumothoraxes, 5 uncomplicated bacterial cellulitis infections, 2 atypical mycobacterial infections requiring multiple debridements, and 18 cases of ulceration necrosis or mastectomy flap necrosis. Most of the authors' cases of skin necrosis occurred in the mid to early portion of their experience as they moved from conservatism to learning the limits of how much fat grafting a recipient site tolerates. For mastectomy patients,

Table 1
Complication rates from the authors' series of 1877 autologous fat transfer procedures performed on 616 breasts of 488 patients over a 6-month to 7-year follow-up period

Category	Radiated Lumpectomy	Immediate Nonradiated	Immediate Radiated	Delayed Nonradiated	Delayed Radiated	Total
Pneumothoraces	1 (1.0%)	1 (1.4%)	0	0	3 (1.9%)	5 (0.8%)
Microbacterial infections	0	0	2 (13%)	0	0	2 (0.3%)
Ulceration necroses	2 (2.0%)	2 (2.8%)	2 (13%)	3 (1.1%)	9 (5.8%)	18 (2.9%)
Locoregional recurrences[3]	2 (2.0%)	0	0	0	1 (0.6%)	3 (0.5%)
Complications[4]	3	3	4	3	12	25
Complication rate per operation	1.5%	2.0%	6.3%	0.4%	1.7%	1.3%

the ulceration rate was significantly greater in radiated breasts (6.5%) than in nonradiated breasts (1.4%) (P<.01). The authors' incidence of pneumothorax was lower than that reported in traditional breast augmentation.[32] When each subset of the patient population was examined, immediate reconstruction patients had better results with fewer procedures than delayed reconstruction patients. Nonradiated patients had better results and fewer complications with fewer procedures than radiated patients. Skin-sparing and nipple-sparing mastectomies had higher complication rates attributed to mastectomy skin flap issues and excess skin, which developed difficult to release folds and adhesions to the chest wall.

Palpable masses developed in 12% of the nonradiated breasts and 37% of radiated breasts. Most of these were oil cysts diagnosed in office by ultrasound and treated by aspiration. Solid masses were worked up by MRI and 32 (5.2%) suspicious lesions were biopsied. Three (0.5%) locoregional recurrences or new primary tumors developed over the 2.5-year mean follow-up period in 2 radiated lumpectomies and 1 mastectomy.

COST ANALYSIS

Taking into account the required revisions and additional fat grafting, cost analysis revealed that unilateral reconstruction with DIEP/TRAM flaps costs $48,058, a 3-stage reconstruction with expanders/implants costs $33,657, whereas even a 4-stage reconstruction with Brava + AFT costs only $22,458. Therefore, without even accounting for the higher rate of costly complications of flaps and implants, breast reconstruction with Brava + AFT is substantially more economical.

DISCUSSION

Tissue engineering consists of seeding biological scaffolds with cells. All currently available implantable scaffolds, however, lack a functional 3D capillary network connected to the host circulation.[33] The authors' finding that Brava external expansion can generate such a scaffold led them to explore and further refine this paradigm shift for breast reconstruction. Instead of the complication-prone flap transfers and implants, the authors use an external device that induces the defect to temporarily generate the required scaffold and then seed it with tissue harvested by simple liposuction (see **Fig. 1**).

Fat grafting is 3D grafting, a novel concept for plastic surgeons more familiar with traditional 2-dimensional skin grafting. Although this requires new conceptual thinking and tools, the principles of graft survival are the same: no tissue can survive more than 2 mm away from the recipient vasculature (graft to recipient interface); and one cannot expect more grafts to survive than what the recipient site can accommodate (recipient size limitation).[11] Fat grafting is akin to sowing seeds in a field. Sowing requires craftsmanship in dispersing the individual seeds to optimize their contact with the soil. Crowding is counterproductive, and harvest yield depends on the size of field and the quality of the soil. Even "superseeds" and "magic grow" additives cannot overcome the limitation of a tiny rocky plot. Numerous additives and fat preparations have failed to convincingly prove better fat survival and thus better, long-term outcomes.[34,35] Without pre-expansion, a mastectomy defect can only accept limited amounts of grafts per session; thus, surgeons attempting to reconstruct an entire breast with AFT alone require a large number of grafting sessions to only achieve moderate breast volumes.[36] The authors attribute much of their success in achieving a long-lasting whole breast reconstruction to a fundamental principle: that large-volume graft survival requires a well-vascularized large-volume recipient scaffold.[11,13]

Breast reconstruction with Brava + AFT is more than just simple fat harvest and reinjection. To obtain the best results, a surgeon needs to be skilled in scar release and expansion using PALF to "melt" away the scars that frequently accompany mastectomy incisions and previously failed breast reconstruction attempts. The important "Rigottomy" (percutaneous needle-meshing maneuver) transforms a restrictive cicatrix into a receptive matrix for the fat grafts.[12,21] The surgeon also needs to recognize "overgrafting" and avoid the temptation to graft more than what the recipient site can safely accommodate. Knowing when to stop fat grafting is the most difficult challenge. For those early in their breast fat-grafting experience, the authors recommend monitoring interstitial fluid pressure via a 14-G needle connected to a standard vascular pressure monitor.

In comparison with published reports of an average of 100 mL of fat transferred per breast in AFT breast reconstruction,[37–40] the authors' mean of 225 mL compares favorably. Indeed, the authors' recent study on cosmetic AFT found that pre-expanded breasts accept a greater volume with a higher retention rate than what is reported in studies on AFT with nonexpanded breasts.[6] Because the authors are able to retain more fat graft volume with each surgical session, the average mastectomy reconstruction required only 2.7 grafting sessions for the nonradiated defects and 4.9 for the radiated sites; this is substantially less than the average 6.5 operations reported for traditional procedures.[41,42]

The authors do not consider percentage graft survival to be a meaningful outcome measure[11]: 50 mL of fat injected into a 500-mL recipient represents only a 10% size increase and almost all of the graft will survive. However, if 500 mL of the same graft preparation is injected into a 50-mL recipient, the size increases 10-fold, the circulation chokes, and the outcome is necrosis. Everything was the same except the graft-to-recipient ratio. The most meaningful outcome is the relative volume gained compared with the size of the original defect. This percentage augmentation of a recipient is the most meaningful index of success in large-volume fat grafting.[13,35]

Complication rates for Brava + AFT breast reconstruction are low. The authors witnessed 2.9% skin ulceration/necrosis, and less than 1% of rate of infection and pneumothorax. Other studies on breast reconstruction with AFT also report low complication rates.[43–45] Most complications occurred in irradiated breast. Radiated breast tissue is less compliant, making overgrafting, and its inherent complications, more likely to occur. Uda and colleagues[45] published a report where they replicated the authors' protocol on 14 patients and produced similar results for nonradiated breasts but concluded that the technique is not suitable for radiated breasts.[46] The authors disagree with the latter finding of Uda and colleagues. Fat grafting to the irradiated breast can reverse radiation damage[14] to yield superior results; however, it requires greater craftsmanship and experience.

An advantage of Brava + AFT breast reconstruction over traditional methods is the ability of the former to preserve, even restore, sensation. Although the authors cannot fully explain why, most of their patients had have near-normal sensation—a stark contrast to cold, insensate implants and poorly sensing flaps. The authors think that this alternative lowers the acceptance threshold for prophylactic mastectomies and hope that it may also sway women to proceed with therapeutic total mastectomies and immediate AFT reconstruction and avoid the late radiation complications associated with lumpectomies.

Overall rate of palpable breast masses was about 19%. Although most were oil cysts and benign scars, and their incidence was not higher than what is commonly seen in other well-accepted breast operations, such as flap reconstructions[47] and breast reductions,[48] one cannot underscore the psychological impact any new detected mass has in the patient with breast cancer. The authors encourage diligent evaluation of the regenerated breast mound and they approach all masses with a high index of suspicion. Recent reviews of AFT to the breast have found no increase in cancer recurrence rates.[49–53] In the authors' 2.5-year follow-up period, 3 locoregional cancer recurrences are predicted in 99 lumpectomy patients; the authors only witnessed 2 recurrences. Furthermore, over this same time frame, only 1 of 389 mastectomy patients developed a locoregional recurrence, while statistics predicted 7 recurrences.[54–56] This reduction is statistically significant. The authors' recurrence rates compare favorably with those observed in reconstruction with flaps and implants,[57] further establishing Brava + AFT as a safe modality of breast reconstruction from a tumorigenesis standpoint.

Cost analysis indicates that Brava + AFT breast reconstruction is substantially less expensive than uncomplicated DIEP/TRAM flap-based reconstructions and tissue expander/implant-based reconstructions. At current breast reconstruction volumes and case mix in the United States, if all breast reconstructions were done with Brava + AFT, health care savings would amount to $1.8 billion dollars annually. This saving is not taking into account the additional high cost of treating complications associated with traditional breast reconstruction.

SUMMARY

There is much more to Brava + AFT breast reconstruction than simple liposuction and reinjection; it is the pre-expansion, the crucial ancillary moves, the craftsmanship in distributing the graft, and the adherence to fundamental principles that makes these remarkable outcomes possible. The authors conclude that the aesthetic quality of the reconstruction, the high patient satisfaction with their sensate breasts, the minimal invasiveness, the low complication rate, and the substantially lower overall costs achieved with this breakthrough tissue engineering breast reconstruction alternative are unmatched.

REFERENCES

1. American Cancer Society. Breast reconstruction after mastectomy. Available at: http://www.cancer.org/acs/groups/cid/documents/webcontent/002992-pdf.pdf. Accessed October 30, 2013.
2. Khouri RK, Rigotti G, Baker TJ. Minimally invasive autologous total breast reconstruction by external expansion and serial lipografting: a preliminary experience. Presented at the 87th Annual Meeting of the American Association of Plastic Surgeons. Boston (MA), April 5–8, 2008.

3. Khouri RK, Eisenmann-Klein M, Cardoso E, et al. Brava and autologous fat transfer is a safe and effective breast augmentation alternative: results of a 6-year, 81-patient, prospective multicenter study. Plast Reconstr Surg 2012;129:1173–87.

4. Khouri RK, Schlenz I, Murphy BJ, et al. Nonsurgical breast enlargement using an external soft-tissue expansion system. Plast Reconstr Surg 2000; 105(7):2500–14.

5. Khouri RK, Del Vecchio D. Breast reconstruction and augmentation using pre-expansion and autologous fat transplantation. Clin Plast Surg 2009;36(2): 269–80.

6. Chin MS, Ogawa R, Lancerotto L, et al. In vivo acceleration of skin growth using a servo-controlled stretching device. Tissue Eng Part C Methods 2010;16(3):397–405.

7. Liu PH, Lew DH, Mayer H, et al. Micro-mechanical forces as a potent stimulator of wound healing. J Am Coll Surg 2004;199:57.

8. Heit YI, Lancerotto L, Mesteri I, et al. External volume expansion increases subcutaneous thickness, cell proliferation, and vascular remodeling in a murine model. Plast Reconstr Surg 2012;130:1–8.

9. Lancerotto L, Chin MS, Freniere B, et al. Mechanisms of action of external volume expansion devices. Plast Reconstr Surg 2013;132(3):569–78.

10. Khouri RK, Rigotti G, Cardoso E, et al. Megavolume autologous fat transfer:– part I. Theory and principles. Plast Reconstr Surg 2014;133(3):550–7.

11. Khouri RK, Khouri RK Jr, Rigotti G, et al. Aesthetic applications of Brava-assisted mega-volume fat grafting to the breasts: a 9-year, 476-patient, multicenter experience. Plast Reconstr Surg 2014; 133(4):796–807.

12. Khouri RK, Rigotti G, Cardoso E, et al. Mega-volume autologous fat transfer: part II. Practice and techniques. Plast Reconstr Surg 2014;133(6):1369–77.

13. Rigotti G, Marchi A, Galie M, et al. Clinical treatment of radiotherapy tissue damage by lipoaspirate transplant: a healing process medicated by adipose-derived adult stem cells. Plast Reconstr Surg 2007;119(5):1409–22.

14. Mojallal A, Lequeux C, Shipkov C, et al. Improvement of skin quality after fat grafting: clinical observation and an animal study. Plast Reconstr Surg 2009;124(3):765–74.

15. Di Summa PG, Kalbermatten DF, Pralong E, et al. Long-term in vivo regeneration of peripheral nerves through bioengineered nerves grafts. Neuroscience 2011;181:278–91.

16. Strassburg S, Nienhusser H, Bjorn Stark G, et al. Co-culture of adipose-derived stem cells and endothelial cells in fibrin induces angiogenesis and vasculogenesis in a chorioallantoic membrane model. J Tissue Eng Regen Med 2013. [Epub ahead of print].

17. Smahel J. Experimental implantation of adipose tissue fragments. Br J Plast Surg 1989;42:207–11.

18. Milosevic MF, Fyles AW, Wong R, et al. Interstitial fluid pressure in cervical carcinoma: within tumor heterogeneity, and relation to oxygen tension. Cancer 1998;82(12):2418–26.

19. Milosevic MF, Fyles AW, Hill RP. The relationship between elevated interstitial fluid pressure and blood flow in tumors: a bioengineering approach. Int J Radiat Oncol Biol Phys 1999;43(5):1111–23.

20. Khouri RK, Smit JM, Cardoso E, et al. Percutaneous aponeurotomy and lipofilling: a regenerative alternative to flap reconstruction? Plast Reconstr Surg 2013;132(5):1280–90.

21. Khouri RK, Cardoso E, Rotemberg S. The reverse abdominoplasty and fat transfer (RAFT) Procedure: A minimally invasive, autologous breast reconstruction alternative. Presented at the 25th Meeting of the European Association of Plastic Surgeons (EURAPS). Isle of Ischia (Italy), May 29–31, 2014.

22. Kovacs L, Eder M, Hollweck R. Comparison between breast volume measurement using 3D surface imaging and classical techniques. Breast 2007;16(2):137–45.

23. Current Procedure Terminology(CPT 2013) copyright 2013 American Medical Association(AMA) All Rights Reserved CPT is a registered trademark of the AMA.

24. National average Medicare payments is calculated using the Conversion Factor of $35.8228 Federal Register Vol. 78, No 237, Part II, December 10, 2013.

25. CMS-1600 FC.42 CFR Parts 405, 410, 411, et al. Revisions to Payment Policies Under the Physician Fee Schedule.

26. Federal Register, Vol 78, No 237, Part III, December 10, 2013.

27. CMS -1601-FC. 42 CFR Parts 405, 410, 411, et al Hospital Outpatient Prospective Payment and Ambulatory Surgical Center Payment Systems.

28. ICD-9-CM Expert for Hospitals and Payers, Volumes 1, 2, 3 Professional Edition 2014. American Medical Association (AMA) Copyright 2013 All Right Reserved.

29. Federal Register, Vol 78, No. 160, Part II, August 19, 2013.

30. CMS - 1599-F; CMS - 1455-F.42 CFR Parts 412, 413, 414, et al. Hospital Inpatient Prospective Payment Systems.

31. Schneider LF, Albornoz CR, Huang J, et al. Incidence of pneumothorax during tissue expander-implant reconstruction and algorithm for intraoperative management. Ann Plast Surg 2013; 0:1–3.

32. Carletti E, Motta A, Migliaresi C. Scaffolds for tissue engineering and 3D cell culture. Methods Mol Biol 2011;695:17–39.

33. Salgarello M, Visconti G, Rusciani A. Breast fat grafting with platelet-rich plasma: a comparative clinical study and current state of the art. Plast Reconstr Surg 2011;127(6):2175–85.

34. Zhao J, Yi C, Zheng Y, et al. Enhancement of fat graft survival by bone marrow-derived mesenchymal stem cell therapy. Plast Reconstr Surg 2013; 132(5):1149–57.

35. Delay E, Garson S, Tousson G, et al. Fat injection to the breast: technique, results, and indications based on 880 procedures over 10 years. Aesthet Surg J 2009;29(5):360–76.

36. Delaporte T, Delay E, Toussoun G, et al. Breast volume reconstruction by lipomodeling technique: about 15 consecutive cases. Ann Chir Plast Esthet 2009;54(4):303–16.

37. Doren EL, Parikh RP, Laronga C, et al. Sequelae of fat grafting postmastectomy: an algorithm for management of fat necrosis. Eplasty 2012;12:e53.

38. Choi M, Small J, Levovitz C, et al. The volumetric analysis of fat graft survival in breast reconstruction. Plast Reconstr Surg 2013;131(2):185–91.

39. Losken A, Pinell XA, Sikoro J, et al. Autologous fat grafting in secondary breast reconstruction. Ann Plast Surg 2011;66(5):518–22.

40. Losken A, Carlson GW, Schoemann MB, et al. Factors that influence the completion of breast reconstruction. Ann Plast Surg 2004;52(3):258–61.

41. Losken A, Nicholas CS, Pinell XA, et al. Outcomes evaluation following bilateral breast reconstruction using latissimus dorsi myocutaneous flaps. Ann Plast Surg 2010;65(1):17–22.

42. Khouri RK, Khouri RK Jr. Percent augmentation: the more meaningful index of success in fat grafting. Plast Reconstr Surg 2015. [Epub ahead of print].

43. Seth AK, Hirsch EM, Kim JY, et al. Long-term outcomes following fat grafting in prosthetic breast reconstruction: a comparative analysis. Plast Reconstr Surg 2012;130(5):984–90.

44. Claro F Jr, Figueiredo JC, Zampar AG, et al. Applicability and safety of autologous fat for reconstruction of the breast. Br J Surg 2012;99(6):768–80.

45. Uda H, Sugawara Y, Sarukawa S, et al. Brava and autologous fat grafting for breast reconstruction after cancer surgery. Plast Reconstr Surg 2013; 133(2):203–13.

46. Casey WJ 3rd, Rebecca AM, Silverman A, et al. Etiology of breast masses after autologous breast reconstruction. Ann Surg Oncol 2013;20(2):607–14.

47. Mandrekas AD, Assimakopoulos GI, Mastorakos DP, et al. Fat necrosis following breast reduction. Br J Plast Surg 1994;47(8):560–2.

48. Fraser JK, Hedrich MH, Cohen SR. Oncologic risks of autologous fat grafting to the breast. Aesthet Surg J 2011;31(1):68–75.

49. Ihrai T, Georgiou C, Machiavello JC. Autologous fat grafting and breast cancer recurrences: retrospective analysis of a series of 100 procedures in 64 patients. J Plast Surg Hand Surg 2013;47(4):273–5.

50. Petit JY, Lohsiriwat V, Clough KB, et al. The oncologic outcome and immediate surgical complications of lipofilling in breast cancer patients: a multicenter study–Milan-Paris-Lyon experience of 646 lipofilling procedures. Plast Reconstr Surg 2011;128(2):341–6.

51. Brenelli F, Rietjens M, De Lorenzi F, et al. Oncological safety of autologous fat grafting after conservative breast treatment: a prospective evaluation. Breast J 2014;20:159–65.

52. Rigotti G, Marchi A, Stringhini P, et al. Determining the oncological risk of autologous lipoaspirate grafting for post-mastectomy breast reconstruction. Aesthetic Plast Surg 2010;34(4):475–80.

53. Fisher B, Anderson S, Bryant J, et al. Twenty-year follow-up of a randomized trial comparing total mastectomy, lumpectomy, and lumpectomy plus irradiation for the treatment of invasive breast cancer. N Engl J Med 2002;347(16):1233–41.

54. Van Dongen JA, Voogd AC, Fentiman IS, et al. Long-term results of a randomized trial comparing breast-conserving therapy with mastectomy: European Organization for Research and Treatment of Cancer 10801 trial. J Natl Cancer Inst 2000;92(14):1143–50.

55. Jacobson JA, Danforth DN, Cowan KH. Ten-year results of a comparison of conservation with mastectomy in the treatment of stage I and II breast cancer. N Engl J Med 1995;332(14):907–11.

56. Liang TJ, Wang BW, Liu SI. Recurrence after skin-sparing mastectomy and immediate transverse rectus abdominis musculocutaneous flap reconstruction for invasive breast cancer. World J Surg Oncol 2013;11(1):194.

57. Van Mierto DR, Penha L, Schipper RJ, et al. No increase of local recurrence rate in breast cancer patients treated with skin-sparing mastectomy followed by immediate breast reconstruction. Breast 2013; 22(6):1168–70.

Safety of Lipofilling in Patients with Breast Cancer

Jean Yves Petit, MD[a],*, Patrick Maisonneuve, Eng[b],
Nicole Rotmensz, MSc[b], Francesco Bertolini, MD, PhD[c],
Krishna Bentley Clough, MD[d], Isabelle Sarfati, MD[d],
Katherine Louise Gale, MD[e], Robert Douglas Macmillan, MD, PhD[f],
Pierre Rey, MD[a,g], Djiazi Benyahi, MD[d], Mario Rietjens, MD[a]

KEYWORDS

- Lipofilling • Fat transfer • Breast cancer • Mastectomy • Breast conservative treatment
- Breast reconstruction • Oncoplasty • Recurrences

KEY POINTS

- Biological considerations: review of experimental research and translational studies.
- Technique: differentiate the transfer technique with simple purification of the fat or an enrichment technique.
- Clinical evaluation based on a reliable statistical method to limit the risk of bias.
- Randomized trial is the best method but is not realistic in plastic surgery indications (patients refuse to submit to the surgeon choice).
- Prospective studies are more reliable than retrospective studies but require long accrual periods.
- Prospective or retrospective studies should at least be case-control studies.
- Definitive conclusions require large series, control groups with a rigorous matching of the cancer criteria, and at least 5 years' mean follow-up.

INTRODUCTION

Lipotransfer represents a technical revolution in plastic surgery and is increasingly used worldwide. Although known for several decades, it is only recently that lipofilling has found a widespread indication in patients with breast cancer to improve the results of breast reconstructions and to correct deformities after conservative treatment. Several publications in the plastic surgery literature underline the technique's versatility and the quality of the results.[1–8] They show the efficacy of lipofilling as a cosmetic procedure, and propose it as a safe, neutral biological material that is able to restore the body contour. Several studies underline the power of transferred fat to regenerate blood supply in skin disorders following radiotherapy.[9,10] Such active regeneration of tissue can be explained by the presence of a high percentage of progenitor cells included in fat tissue.[11] In this regard, attention must be drawn to the recent and abundant preclinical studies that show that adipose progenitor cells may promote breast cancer growth and metastasis. As recent studies have shown, white adipose tissue

[a] Division of Plastic and Reconstructive Surgery, European Institute of Oncology, Milan 20141, Italy; [b] Division of Epidemiology and Biostatistics, European Institute of Oncology, Milan 20141, Italy; [c] Division of Laboratory Haematology-Oncology, European Institute of Oncology, Milan 20141, Italy; [d] Institut du Sein, Paris 75016, France; [e] Division of Oncoplastic Surgery, Waitemata DHB, Auckland, New Zealand; [f] Division of Oncoplastic Surgery, Nottingham Breast Institute, Nottingham NG51PB, UK; [g] Centro di Senologia, Genolier Swiss Medical Network, Lugano, Switzerland
* Corresponding author. Division of Plastic and Reconstructive Surgery, European Institute of Oncology, Via Ripamonti 435, Milan 20141, Italy.
E-mail address: jean.petit@ieo.it

Clin Plastic Surg 42 (2015) 339–344
http://dx.doi.org/10.1016/j.cps.2015.03.004
0094-1298/15/$ – see front matter © 2015 Elsevier Inc. All rights reserved.

(WAT)–derived progenitor cells can contribute to tumor vessels, pericytes, and adipocytes, and were found to stimulate local and metastatic progression of breast cancer in several murine models.[12–14] Experimental studies provide data on the endocrine, paracrine, and autocrine activity of the transplanted fat tissue.[15] Adipocyte, preadipocyte, and progenitor cell production of adipokines and several other secretions can stimulate angiogenesis and growth of breast cancerous cells.[16] This tumor-stroma interaction can potentially induce cancer reappearance by fueling dormant breast cancer cells in the tumor bed.[17] A case report describes a local recurrence more than 13 years after apparent cure of an osteosarcoma, 1 year after lipofilling of the shoulder for cosmetic repair.[18] Moreover a case-control study revealed a significant increase of local recurrences in patients with intraepithelial breast neoplasia who underwent a lipofilling procedure for breast reconstruction.[19,20]

Concern about radiologic sequelae and surveillance difficulties by mammography caused by lipofilling has been addressed in the literature, particularly with regard to the risk of calcifications observed after lipofilling affecting the diagnosis of recurrences. This issue has largely been resolved by the distinction between suspicious fine, linear, and pleomorphic microcalcifications, and macrocalcifications related to fat necrosis as observed in most cases after fat transfer.[3,21,22]

In order to confirm the safety of lipofilling procedures in patients with breast cancer, clinical studies based on adequate statistical method and accurate follow-up are required to show that the local recurrence rate, as well as any cancer event, is not increased in fat-grafted patients with breast cancer.

BIOLOGICAL CONSIDERATIONS

There is increasing evidence that obesity, an excess accumulation of adipose tissue occurring when caloric intake exceeds energy expenditure, is associated with an increased frequency and morbidity of several types of neoplastic diseases, including postmenopausal breast cancer. Disruption of the energy homeostasis results in obesity, inflammation, and alterations of adipokine signaling that may foster initiation and progression of cancer.[23–25] Preclinical studies have suggested that differentiated cells of the WAT and WAT-resident progenitors may also promote cancer growth and metastasis. We described that CD45-CD34+ progenitors from human WAT may promote breast cancer growth and metastases in preclinical models.[13] Other recent studies, some of which are based on endogenous WAT expressing

a transgenic reporter, showed a significant level of adipose cell contribution to tumor composition. However, WAT contains several distinct populations of progenitors, and these data were obtained using crude or mixed cell populations. We therefore decided to purify by sorting the 2 quantitatively most relevant populations of WAT progenitors (endothelial progenitor cells [EPCs] and adipose stromal cells) and to investigate, in vitro and in vivo, their roles in several orthotopic models of local and metastatic breast cancer. One study has recently described that EPCs are present in tissues other than the bone marrow, in particular in the adipose tissue of mice. This article reports that human WAT is a rich reservoir of CD45-CD34+ EPCs.[11] Compared with bone marrow-derived CD34+ cells mobilized in blood by granulocyte colony–stimulating factor, purified human WAT-derived CD34+ cells were found to express similar levels of stemness-related genes and significantly increased levels of angiogenesis-related genes and of fibroblast activation protein alpha (FAP-α), which is a crucial suppressor of antitumor immunity.[26] In vitro, WAT-CD34+ cells generated mature endothelial cells and endothelial tubes. In vivo, the coinjection of human WAT-CD34+ cells contributed to orthotopic tumor vascularization and significantly increased tumor growth and metastasis in models of human breast cancer in nonobese, diabetic, severe combined immunodeficient interleukin-2 receptor gamma–null mice.

LIPOFILLING TECHNIQUES

Two procedures should be differentiated according to the technique of lipofilling: the simple purification of the liposuction specimen and the enrichment of adipose tissue–derived stromal cells (ADSCs). The first, the so-called Coleman technique, does not modify the concentration of ADSCs, and the second, the so-called enrichment technique, increases the concentration of the ADSCs in the specimen that will be used for the reconstruction. In the Coleman technique[27] the fat tissue is obtained by liposuction performed on a fatty area of the body (abdomen or thighs). The specimen is purified by soft centrifugation to discard the oil and blood cells. Then the purified fat is injected in the area to be reshaped. Small differences of technique are proposed to purify the specimen without modifying the concentration of ADSCs. The main drawback of this technique is the frequency of reabsorption of the fat tissue injected in the following 6 months.[28,29] In contrast, the enrichment technique divides the specimen obtained by liposuction into 2 parts. The first part is reserved for the final injection. The second is processed in a machine using an enzymatic procedure (with a collagenase) to destroy the adult adipocytes and concentrate the ADSCs. The small amount of concentrated progenitor cells obtained by this procedure is then mixed with the first reserved specimen. The enriched fat tissue is then used for reshaping the breast.[8] Promoters of the enrichment technique argue that the ADSCs' concentration favors the regenerative process of the recipient tissues and decreases the risk of reabsorption of the fat tissue injected in the Coleman technique.[30]

PUBLISHED CLINICAL STUDIES IN PATIENTS WITH BREAST CANCER

In a first study conducted at the European Institute of Oncology (IEO),[19] the outcome of 321 patients with breast cancer who received lipofilling to improve the results of a reconstruction after partial or total mastectomy was compared with that of a matched control group of 642 patients who did not receive lipofilling. No statistical difference between the local recurrence rates of the two groups was observed (hazard ratio [HR], 1.1; 95% confidence interval [CI], 0.47–2.64; $P = .79$). In subgroup analyses, no difference in local recurrence rate was observed for the types of breast surgery (breast conservative procedure or mastectomy) but a difference was observed for patients with intraepithelial neoplasia. Because of the small size of this group, no definitive conclusion was drawn.[19]

To better investigate the potential risk of local recurrence in women with intraepithelial neoplasia, a successive study was performed focused on a larger group of 59 patients with intraepithelial-only breast cancer who received lipofilling.[20] This group was compared with a matched control group of 118 patients who did not receive lipofilling. Again, the local recurrence rate was significantly higher in the study group than in the control group (HR, 4.5; 95% CI, 1.1–18.2; $P = .02$).

Although there was no apparent explanation for such increased risk of recurrence in women with intraepithelial neoplasia, we published our results to raise an alert and stimulate further studies on independent larger series and possibly longer follow-up.[19,20]

STUDIES IN MILAN AND PARIS

First, we repeated the analysis of our study in women with intraepithelial neoplasia after a longer period of follow-up, allowing for more events to occur in both the study and the control groups. In order to limit the number of patients lost at follow-up, patients no longer attending follow-up visits at our institute were individually contacted by a clinician and information on their status and outcome was recorded. Second, we compared our updated results with those (K.B. Clough, unpublished, 2014) observed in a similar series of 48 patients with intraepithelial neoplasia treated with fat transfer at the Institut du Sein in Paris, France.

The annual local recurrence rate was 2.8% in the lipofilling group in Milan and 1.5% in the lipofilling group in Paris compared with 1.2% in the control group in Milan, with no statistically significant difference in the recurrence rates between groups (lipofilling/Milan vs lipofilling/Paris, $P = .40$; lipofilling/Milan vs control/Milan, $P = .08$; lipofilling/Paris vs control/Milan, $P = .81$). Data from patients who received lipofilling in Milan and Paris were pooled and, again, we did not observe a statistically significant difference in breast cancer recurrence compared with the Milan control group ($P = .14$) (**Table 1**).

We then evaluated separately the outcome of patients who underwent breast-conserving surgery and those who underwent mastectomy. The recurrence rate was similar in the lipofilling group and the control group of women who had

Table 1
Cumulative incidence of local events in women with intraepithelial breast neoplasia who received lipofilling (59 from Milan, 48 from Paris) and in a group of 118 controls matched to the Milan cases

Study	Group	Patients	Local Recurrences	Patient-years	Rate/100 y
			Cumulative Incidence of Local Recurrence (%)		
Milan	Lipofilling	59	8	285	2.8
Paris	Lipofilling	48	2	130	1.5
Milan plus Paris	Lipofilling	107	10	415	2.4
Milan	Matched control	118	8	679	1.2
Lazzeroni et al,[31] 2013	Unmatched control[a]	1171	163	NA	2.1

Abbreviation: NA, not available.
[a] Consecutive series of patients with ductal intraepithelial neoplasia unselected for having received or not received breast reconstruction, with or without lipofilling.

mastectomy ($P = .56$). It was higher in the lipofilling group than in the control group of women who had breast-conserving surgery, but the excess was not statistically significant ($P = .20$) (**Table 2**).

STUDY IN NOTTINGHAM

Gale and Macmillan in Nottingham (United Kingdom) performed a case-control study with a design similar to the Milan study: 211 patients with breast cancer receiving lipofilling were compared with 422 matched controls. No statistical difference was observed between the recurrence rate of the study group and the control group for local recurrence rate (0.95% vs 1.90%; $P = .33$), regional recurrence rate (0.95% vs 0%; $P = .16$), and distant recurrence rate (3.32% vs 2.61%; $P = .65$). Among the 211 cases, only 27 were intraepithelial and no locoregional recurrence was observed in this group. Macmillan concluded that "no evidence of increased oncologic risk was associated with fat grafting in women previously treated for breast cancer."[32]

DISCUSSION

The 3 studies in Milan, Paris, and Nottingham are similar with regard to the technique of lipofilling, all of them using the Coleman technique. The Nottingham investigators analyzed their results after lipotransfer in patients with breast cancer in a

case-control study.[32] No increase in the number of local recurrences in the intraepithelial neoplasia group was observed but the number of cases in this series was probably too small to show a difference. We previously observed an excess rate of recurrences in patients with intraepithelial neoplasia who received lipofilling in the Milan study, but the difference could have been caused by the unexpected low recurrence rate in the control group, and could therefore be the result of chance. In a repeat analysis, after a longer follow-up period the observed difference was no more statistically significant, because more recurrences were reported in the control group during the updated follow-up time. The recurrence rate in the Paris study was similar to that in the Milan study. However, the Paris study lacked a matched control group, and we could only make a comparison with the control group from Milan.

When we combined the cases of the 3 studies dealing with the Coleman technique, in order to increase statistical power, no significant increase of local recurrence was observed. The strength of the Milan studies and the Nottingham study is the quality of the comparison using precise case match criteria. One of the difficulties in matching the populations was the risk of bias caused by the great variation in lapse time between the primary surgery (cancer treatment) and the date of lipofilling. The study population was selected among the patients who did not have a cancer

Table 2
Cumulative incidence of local events in women with intraepithelial breast neoplasia who received lipofilling (59 from Milan, 48 from Paris) and in a group of 118 controls matched to the Milan cases according to type of surgery

Study	Group	Patients	Local Recurrences	Patient-years	Rate/100 y
			Cumulative Incidence of Local Recurrence (%)		
Breast-conserving Surgery					
Milan	Lipofilling	12	3	52	5.8
Paris	Lipofilling	9	0	21	0.0
Milan plus Paris	Lipofilling	21	3	73	4.1
Milan	Matched control	25	2	140	1.4
Lazzeroni et al,[31] 2013	Unmatched control[a]	872	142	NA	2.5
Mastectomy					
Milan	Lipofilling	47	5	233	2.1
Paris	Lipofilling	39	2	109	1.8
Milan plus Paris	Lipofilling	86	7	342	2.0
Milan	Matched control	93	6	540	1.1
Lazzeroni et al,[31] 2013	Unmatched control[a]	299	21	NA	1.1

[a] Consecutive series of patients with ductal intraepithelial neoplasia unselected for having received or not received breast reconstruction, with or without lipofilling.

event during this lapse time. Because the lipofilled patients received their fat transfers at different times after the initial cancer treatment and the length of the disease-free period modifies the local recurrence risk after the lipofilling, it was necessary to match the controls according to the length of the different lapse times between primary surgery and lipofilling. The weakness of these studies is the population size of the intraepithelial cancers: 59 patients in the Milan study, 48 in the Paris study, and 27 in the Nottingham study. The short follow-up of the series was also an important limitation: around 2 years after the lipofilling. The last review of the Milan study showed a disappearance of the significant difference. In addition, the rate of local relapse in our series of patients who received lipofilling is similar to that reported in a large series of 1171 consecutive patients treated for ductal intraepithelial neoplasia in a single institution (IEO) unselected for having received or not received breast reconstruction, with or without lipofilling.[31]

In a systematic review on the safety of autologous lipoaspirate grafting in patients with breast cancer, Krastev and colleagues[33] reviewed 394 articles dealing with fat transfer. After selection according to the content of cancer data, the quality of the follow-up, and the size of the series, the investigators found only 9 articles fulfilling the cancer criteria requirements. Among these 9 articles, they found no prospective study and no randomized trials. Only 2 retrospective studies had a control group. One by Rigotti and colleagues[10] compared the local recurrence rate of 133 mastectomy cases with lipofilling during the prelipofilling and postlipofilling periods. No increase was observed and Rigotti and colleagues[10] concluded that lipofilling is a safe procedure in patients with cancer, arguing that if lipofilling were detrimental oncologically the rate of recurrences after lipofilling would have been increased. Two criticisms have been made concerning the statistical methodology of this study.[34] One was the exclusion of patients who had breast conservative treatments, which convey a higher risk of residual cancer cells in the breast. The second deals with the methodology: the comparison between local recurrence rates before and after lipofilling can be reliable only if the rate of local recurrence after the primary surgery is constant. However, it is usually stated that the rate of recurrence is higher in the first 5 years and then reaches a plateau. In addition, Krastev and colleagues[33] concluded that, "Whether lipoaspirate grafting promotes local recurrence in breast cancer patients is still unclear. To answer this question, larger prospective trials with longer follow-up are needed." Other reviews also concluded that further prospective studies

are needed to confirm the safety of lipofilling in patients with breast cancer.[35–38]

It is important for more oncologic results to be obtained after using the enrichment technique. Analysis of the literature has shown that, if there is an association between lipofilling and cancer recurrence, then progenitor cells are most likely to be responsible for this by stimulation of remaining cancer cells. These cells are concentrated in the enrichment technique. We did not find any reliable studies showing the safety of enriched lipofilling in patients with breast cancer. The only study reporting cancer outcome, The Restore Study published in 2012, did not find any recurrence in the series of 67 patients after a follow-up of 1 year. The study was limited by the size of the study group, the lack of controls, and the short follow-up.[39]

REFERENCES

1. Ersek RA, Chang P, Salisbury MA. Lipo layering of autologous fat: an improved technique with promising results. Plast Reconstr Surg 1998;101:820–6.
2. Khouri R, Del Vecchio D. Breast reconstruction and augmentation using pre-expansion and autologous fat transplantation. Clin Plast Surg 2009;36:269–80.
3. Report on autologous fat transplantation. ASPRS Ad-Hoc Committee on New Procedures, September 30, 1987. Plast Surg Nurs 1987;7:140–1.
4. Coleman SR. Long-term survival of fat transplants: controlled demonstrations. Aesthetic Plast Surg 1995;19:421–5.
5. Coleman S. Structural fat grafting. St Louis (MO): Quality Medical Publishing; 2004.
6. Delay E, Garson S, Tousson G, et al. Fat injection to the breast: technique, results, and indications based on 880 procedures over 10 years. Aesthet Surg J 2009;29:360–76.
7. Spear SL, Wilson HB, Lockwood MD. Fat injection to correct contour deformities in the reconstructed breast. Plast Reconstr Surg 2005;116:1300–5.
8. Yoshimura K, Sato K, Aoi N, et al. Cell-assisted lipotransfer for cosmetic breast augmentation: supportive use of adipose-derived stem/stromal cells. Aesthetic Plast Surg 2008;32:48–55.
9. Coleman SR. Structural fat grafting: more than a permanent filler. Plast Reconstr Surg 2006;118(3S): 108S–20S.
10. Rigotti G, Marchi A, Stringhini P, et al. Determining the oncological risk of autologous lipoaspirate grafting for post-mastectomy breast reconstruction. Aesthetic Plast Surg 2010;34:475–80.
11. Martin-Padura I, Gregato G, Marighetti P, et al. The white adipose tissue used in lipotransfer procedures is a rich reservoir of CD34+ progenitors able to promote cancer progression. Cancer Res 2012;72:325–34.

12. Zhang Y, Daquinag A, Traktuev DO, et al. White adipose tissue cells are recruited by experimental tumors and promote cancer progression in mouse models. Cancer Res 2009;69:5259–66.

13. Orecchioni S, Gregato G, Martin-Padura I, et al. Complementary populations of human adipose CD34+ progenitor cells promote growth, angiogenesis, and metastasis of breast cancer. Cancer Res 2013;73:5880–91.

14. Rowan BG, Gimble JM, Sheng M, et al. Human adipose tissue-derived stromal/stem cells promote migration and early metastasis of triple negative breast cancer xenografts. PLoS One 2014;9: e89595.

15. Park J, Euhus DM, Scherer PE. Paracrine and endocrine effects of adipose tissue on cancer development and progression. Endocr Rev 2011;32:550–70.

16. Wang YY, Lehuédé C, Laurent V, et al. Adipose tissue and breast epithelial cells: a dangerous dynamic duo in breast cancer. Cancer Lett 2012;324: 142–51.

17. Lohsiriwat V, Curigliano G, Rietjens M, et al. Autologous fat transplantation in patients with breast cancer: "silencing" or "fueling" cancer recurrence? Breast 2011;20:351–7.

18. Perrot P, Rousseau J, Bouffaut AL, et al. Safety concern between autologous fat graft, mesenchymal stem cell and osteosarcoma recurrence. PLoS One 2010;5:e10999.

19. Petit JY, Botteri E, Lohsiriwat V, et al. Locoregional recurrence risk after lipofilling in breast cancer patients. Ann Oncol 2012;23:582–8.

20. Petit JY, Rietjens M, Botteri E, et al. Evaluation of fat grafting safety in patients with intraepithelial neoplasia: a matched-cohort study. Ann Oncol 2013;24:1479–84.

21. Pulagam SR, Poulton T, Mamounas EP. Long-term clinical and radiologic results with autologous fat transplantation for breast augmentation: case reports and review of the literature. Breast J 2006; 12:63–5.

22. Veber M, Tourasse C, Toussoun G, et al. Radiographic findings after breast augmentation by autologous fat transfer. Plast Reconstr Surg 2001;127: 1289–99.

23. Bellows CF, Zhang Y, Chen J, et al. Circulation of progenitor cells in obese and lean colorectal cancer patients. Cancer Epidemiol Biomarkers Prev 2011; 20:2461–8.

24. Bellows CF, Zhang Y, Simmons PJ, et al. Influence of BMI on level of circulating progenitor cells. Obesity 2011;19:1722–6.

25. Bertolini F, Orecchioni S, Petit JY, et al. Obesity, proinflammatory mediators, adipose tissue progenitors, and breast cancer. Curr Opin Oncol 2014;26: 545–50.

26. Ouchi N, Parker JL, Lugus JJ, et al. Adipokines in inflammation and metabolic disease. Nat Rev Immunol 2011;11:85–97.

27. Coleman SR, Saboeiro AP. Fat grafting to the breast revisited: safety and efficacy. Plast Reconstr Surg 2007;119:775–85.

28. Peer LA. Loss of weight and volume in human fat grafts: with postulation of a "cell survival theory". Plast Reconstr Surg 1950;5:217–30.

29. Beck M, Amar O, Bodin F, et al. Evaluation of breast lipofilling after sequelae of conservative treatment for cancer. Eur J Plast Surg 2012;35:221–8.

30. Kølle SF, Fischer-Nielsen A, Mathiasen AB, et al. Enrichment of autologous fat grafts with ex-vivo expanded adipose tissue-derived stem cells for graft survival: a randomised placebo-controlled trial. Lancet 2013;382:1113–20.

31. Lazzeroni M, Guerrieri-Gonzaga A, Botteri E, et al. Tailoring treatment for ductal intraepithelial neoplasia of the breast according to Ki-67 and molecular phenotype. Br J Cancer 2013;108: 1593–601.

32. Gale K, Rahka E, Ball G, et al. A case controlled study of the oncological safety of fat grafting. Plast Reconstr Surg, in press.

33. Krastev TK, Jonasse Y, Kon M. Oncological safety of autologous lipoaspirate grafting in breast cancer patients: a systematic review. Ann Surg 2013;20: 111–9.

34. De Lorenzi F, Lohsiriwat V, Petit JY. In response to: Rigotti G, Marchi A, Stringhini P et al. "Determining the oncological risk of autologous lipoaspirate grafting for post-mastectomy breast reconstruction". Aesth Plast Surg 2010;34:475. Aesthetic Plast Surg 2011;35:132–3.

35. Chan CW, McCulley SJ, Macmillan RD. Autologous fat transfer–a review of the literature with a focus on breast cancer surgery. J Plast Reconstr Aesth Surg 2008;61:1438–48.

36. Kling RE, Mehrara BJ, Pusic AL, et al. Trends in autologous fat grafting to the breast: a national survey of the American Society of Plastic Surgeons. Plast Reconstr Surg 2013;132:35–46.

37. Largo RD, Tchang LA, Mele V, et al. Efficacy, safety and complications of autologous fat grafting to healthy breast tissue: a systematic review. J Plast Reconstr Aesth Surg 2013;67:437–48.

38. Rosing JH, Wong G, Wong MS, et al. Autologous fat grafting for primary breast augmentation: a systematic review. Aesthetic Plast Surg 2011;35: 882–90.

39. Pérez-Cano R, Vranckx JJ, Lasso JM, et al. Prospective trial of adipose-derived regenerative cell (ADRC)-enriched fat grafting for partial mastectomy defects: the RESTORE-2 trial. Eur J Surg Oncol 2012;38:382–9.

Regenerative Approach to Scars, Ulcers and Related Problems with Fat Grafting

Marco Klinger, MD[a],*, Andrea Lisa, MD[a], Francesco Klinger, MD[b],
Silvia Giannasi, MD[a], Alessandra Veronesi, MD[a], Barbara Banzatti, MD[a],
Valeria Bandi, MD[a], Barbara Catania, MD[a], Davide Forcellini, MD[b],
Luca Maione, MD[a], Valeriano Vinci, MD[a], Fabio Caviggioli, MD[b]

KEYWORDS

- Autologous fat graft • Scar treatment • Chronic ulcer • Regenerative potential
- Angiographic needles

KEY POINTS

- Autologous fat graft is an innovative surgical option for scars and ulcers that achieves tissue regeneration and remodeling without the need for new and even worse scarring.
- Autologous fat graft is an option of choice in case of wide nonlinear scars, in tension areas, or in cases of depressed scars.
- Experience suggests fat grafting effectiveness in treating chronic skin ulcer of small to moderate size, not exceeding 3.5 cm².
- The use of needles (18-gauge angiographic) is fundamental to treat fibrotic scar tissue. They allow one to perform a highly precise technique, overcoming tissue resistance.
- Fat processing with centrifugation increases adipose-derived stem cell content and reduces the amount of proinflammatory blood cells, maximizing regenerative properties.

 Video of adipose tissue harvesting by infiltration accompanies this article at http://www.plasticsurgery.theclinics.com/

INTRODUCTION

Adipose tissue is a connective tissue containing a reservoir of mesenchymal stem cells that can divide indefinitely, producing various cellular lines.[1–3]

Coleman's[4,5] processing and harvesting technique described in 1992 increased fat graft survival, making its adoption more reliable and predictable. Initially used as a filler to correct volume deficiencies and for esthetic purposes, autologous fat grafting

No financial support or benefits have been received by any author. We have no relationship with any commercial source that is related directly or indirectly to the scientific work. Devices used in this study: Coleman's original kit for lipostructure and 18G needle, Cordis®, a Johnson & Johnson Company, N.V, 9301 LJ, Roden, Netherlands.
[a] Plastic Surgery Unit, Department of Medical Biotechnology and Translational Medicine BIOMETRA, Humanitas Clinical and Research Center, Reconstructive and Aesthetic Plastic Surgery School, University of Milan, Via Manzoni 56, Rozzano, Milan 20089, Italy; [b] Plastic Surgery Unit, Reconstructive and Aesthetic Plastic Surgery School, MultiMedica Holding S.p.A., University of Milan, Via Milanese, 300, Sesto San Giovanni, Milan 20099, Italy
* Corresponding author.
E-mail address: Marco.klinger@humanitas.it

Clin Plastic Surg 42 (2015) 345–352
http://dx.doi.org/10.1016/j.cps.2015.03.008
0094-1298/15/$ – see front matter © 2015 Elsevier Inc. All rights reserved.

has found a progressively greater field of application, and recently has entered regenerative medicine. The experience of Rigotti and coworkers[6] in treating radiodystrophic outcomes obtaining local improvement of tegument trophic characteristics after autologous fat grafting was pioneering.

Inspired by these results, we applied the same technique to burn scars with excellent clinical results. Histologic examination of the treated skin showed patterns of new collagen deposition, local hypervascularity, and dermal hyperplasia with tissue regeneration.[7] Building on these results, we began to treat other kinds of pathologic scars with an overall improvement in tissue quality. In our experience, autologous fat graft has proved to be an efficient and safe procedure to treat scars of different origin, demonstrating the capability of lipostructure to achieve architectural remodeling and loose connective regeneration.[8–14]

In different clinical settings, we observed how lipostructure managed to relieve neuropathic pain thanks not only to regenerative effects, but also as a result of molecular changes induced in the microenvironment and secretion of substances able to give prolonged analgesia.[15–22] Finally, we positively adopted its regenerative properties in the setting of posttraumatic "hard-to-heal" wounds, obtaining an improvement of healed skin quality and elasticity that appears very similar to normal skin.[23,24]

Our clinical experience shows that autologous fat grafting can be adopted in different clinical settings by evolving reconstructive into regenerative surgery. It is well known that scars of different origin may impede function, especially in cases of joint involvement, which may cause discomfort, tightness, or even pain, and achieve cosmetic deformity. Several surgical approaches to treat scar tissue have been described, such as surgical excision and resuturing, Z-plasty, W-plasty, and geometric broken line suturing. However, all these revision techniques are adopted in selected cases and may achieve suboptimal results.

Skin ulcer can be extremely challenging to approach. Treatment is typically to avoid ulcer infection, remove any excess discharge, maintain a moist wound environment, control the edema, and ease pain caused by nerve and tissue damage. Although all these procedures are followed, ulcers do not frequently re-epithelize, showing a tendency to become chronic. This tendency is caused by several factors, such as anatomic location and patient condition, concomitant pathologies, drug assumption, previous local therapy, and smoking.

This article describes how autologous fat grafting regenerative properties can be applied in scar tissue and ulcer treatment.

TREATMENT GOALS AND PLANNED OUTCOMES

In scar tissue–related problems and chronic ulcer, a proper assessment and adequate counseling before treatment are fundamental so that the patient is informed about the expected outcome. We indicate scar treatment with autologous fat graft in cases of wide nonlinear scars, in tension areas, or in cases of depressed scars. We propose treatment only on mature scars, giving a minimum threshold of 2 years from the causative factor. In all these clinical conditions surgical revision could result in a new and even worse scar than the previous one, whereas autologous fat graft and its regenerative properties are the more innovative surgical option.

Patients should be informed that their scars cannot disappear and the purpose of the procedure is local amelioration. Treatment goals include an increase in softness, flexibility, and extensibility of treated tissue with a release of scar bundles in superficial and deep planes, which can favor an improvement of mobility of the body district involved.

In the facial district treatment allows a partial restoration of facial mimic (kiss, smile, and other mood expression) because of the release of scar retraction. In cases of great skin depression a refill of these volume deficits can be obtained. In addition, pain symptoms related to scars can be reduced.

Patients should be informed that, after the first procedure, the result can be partial because of permanence of scar tissue retraction and depression. To obtain a satisfactory final result several procedures may be needed especially in more severe cases. Each procedure should be performed at least 3 months after the previous one to let fat graft manifest its regenerative effects. In some cases, scar release and local improvement can achieve a reduction of skin tension, allowing a secondary surgical scar revision.

In chronic ulcer, our experience suggests fat grafting effectiveness in treating areas of small to moderate size, not exceeding 3.5 cm². For bigger ulcer a combined approach with advanced dressing is needed. We treat posttraumatic ulcers that do not respond to advanced dressings. We are currently widening our indication to ulcers of different causes.

The aim of the treatment is to enhance the wound healing process relying on fat graft regenerative effects, obtaining a complete recovery of tissue integrity. Final re-epithelization can be obtained after more than a single procedure. As for scar treatment, pain symptoms related to ulcers, which highly affect patients' quality of life, can be improved.

PREOPERATIVE PLANNING AND PREPARATION

All patients selected for autologous fat graft procedure need a clinical assessment and routine preoperative examination. In case of scar treatment, preoperative markings are performed, asking the patient to note areas of greater tension and impairment to daily life activities and movements. In case of ulcer treatment, perilesional skin is marked.

Donor areas are abdomen and/or trochanteric and flank areas, given the easier access to abundant amounts of adipose tissue. Donor site is chosen according to the amount of adipose tissue, if previous surgery has been made, and according to patient preference. The areas are generally not marked before surgery.

PROCEDURAL APPROACH

The patient is placed lying down, prone or supine according scar location. Surgical procedure is performed under local anesthesia and sedation assisted with sterile technique. We proceed to infiltration of the donor areas using a blunt cannula filled with anesthetic solution (100 mL saline solution, 10 mL of levobupivacaine 7.5 mg/mL, 20 mL of mepivacaine 10 mg/mL, and 0.5 mL epinephrine 1 mg/mL). Infiltration provides good hemostasis and adequate operative and perioperative analgesic action (Video 1).

Adipose tissue is harvested through the same incision by infiltration of anesthetic solution, with blunt cannulas of 2 to 3 mm in diameter of variable length (between 15 and 23 cm). The cannula used for sampling is connected with a Luer-lock syringe of 10 mL. The syringe plunger is pulled at the top and secured by hand. This creates inside the syringe a slight negative pressure, which allows the levy of adipose tissue while the cannula is advanced and retracted with radial movements inside the donor area (Video 2). When full, the syringe is placed in a centrifuge with resterilized containers and adipose tissue is centrifuged at 3000 rpm for 3 minutes.

Following centrifugation three distinct layers are obtained; only the intermediate one is needed for therapeutic purposes. In our experience centrifugation following the Coleman technique is the ideal processing method to obtain a final product purified and enriched with higher regenerative properties. We have recently demonstrated[25] that centrifugation does not impair cell viability, increasing the content of adipose-derived stem cells and reducing the amount of proinflammatory blood cells. Centrifugation concentrates a higher number of viable cells with regenerative potential in a smaller amount of inoculum, thus making this method ideal for the treatment of retracting scar tissue and ulcers.

Fat is transferred from a 10-mL syringe into a 1-mL syringe Luer-lock that allows precise control of the amount of injected fat and better handling. The adipocyte fraction is injected using an 18-gauge angiographic needle with a snap-on wing (Cordis®; Johnson & Johnson, Roden, the Netherlands). The use of needles is fundamental to treat scar tissue.[24] In our clinical experience, blunt cannulas are not the ideal instruments to perform a quick, safe, and painless procedure and better results are achieved with sharp angiographic needles.

Over the years we have found that scar tissue derived from any factor is characterized by overflowing fibrous tissue that achieves a significant resistance to the sliding of the cannulas used for fat injection. Through an 18-gauge angiographic needle,[26] we are able to perform a highly precise technique, overcoming tissue resistance related to the presence of fibrous tissue, thus making it possible to lay a constant amount of fat at the dermal-hypodermal junction by multiple radiating passages that distribute fat in all directions, creating an ideal web to support damaged areas (Videos 3 and 4).

Lysis of scar tissue is obtained by two different methods. The first consists of pushing the plunger of the syringe and exploiting the strength of exiting fat to overcome the fibrous tissue resistance. In the second method we adopt a retrograde technique entering the needle for its entire length at the dermal-epidermal junction and then, while extracting the needle, releasing fat.

We believe that sharp cannula stimulates new collagen deposition and remodeling of fibrous tissues, in a fashion similar to the "needling" procedure used in aesthetic medicine. Moreover, 18-gauge angiographic sharp needles are disposable and low-cost devices compared with classic blunt cannulas.

The amount of injected fat at each passage is minimized to avoid irregularities and clusters, which are eventually deleted with digital manipulation after the procedure.

POTENTIAL COMPLICATIONS AND THEIR MANAGEMENT

We consider autologous fat grafting to be a safe procedure with a low rate of immediate and late complications at the local and systemic levels. We have recently reviewed our case series after 1000 patients treated[27] and we found no cases of intraoperative complications, such as perforation of abdominal viscera, cardiac arrest, stroke, major bleeding, and death. We report only one case of breast implant rupture in a patient who had undergone previous mastectomy and radiotherapy. We did not find any cases of postoperative systemic complications, such as pulmonary embolism, sepsis, deep venous thrombosis, and mortality.

As to local complications, we had among possible early donor-site complications only two hematomas and also recorded 83 cases of fibrosis (local deformation caused by fat harvesting, <2 cm in diameter) as late donor-site complications. In the recipient site, four cases of infection were noted, and no skin necrosis was observed.

Our main concern related to the use of sharp needles is to provoke intravascular fat injection. Risk can be easily avoided by choosing the retrograde injection method. In our clinical experience, using angiographic needles, we found that edema and bleeding of treated areas have been comparable with those detected using the standard technique, which are virtually nil. Hematomas in the donor site in our experience can be managed with local compression.

Local deformities are more challenging to address. In our experience, we observed only moderate cases, which could be treated with local massage to reduce deep fibrosis and improve contour appearance. In three cases we treated, patients presented severe local deformity after surgery with autologous fat grafting to correct contour defect. To prevent this complication, special caution should be taken when harvesting adipose tissue to perform many radial movements in an overall wide area without passing repeatedly in the same place and thus causing contour defect.

POSTPROCEDURAL CARE

The treated area is covered with a dressing for 1 week and the patient is instructed to avoid pressure and friction to limit fat displacement. The access incisions in the donor areas are sutured with 4/0 Vicryl. Donor areas are managed with an elastic-compressive dressing, which has to be kept in place for 5 days to prevent hematoma formation.

REHABILITATION AND RECOVERY

Patients are discharged on the same day of the operation. Normal activities of daily life and work can be resumed on the first day after operation. Sport activities should be interrupted for 7 days postoperative.

OUTCOMES

In our experience autologous fat grafting has revealed an innovative therapeutic efficacy in the treatment of scars and ulcers as a result of its regenerative effects. Several surgical procedures, such as traditional Z-plasty, dermoepidermal grafts, V-Y flaps, and other local flaps are currently in use to correct scars, together with common medical and conservative procedures, such as elastic-compressive garments, topical silicone sheets, physiotherapy, splints, corticosteroid injection, laser therapy, cryotherapy, and radiotherapy. All of these procedures may obtain positive but partial results.

In the scenario where medical and surgical therapies seem to be ineffective especially in the long term, autologous fat graft and its regenerative properties has proved to be a new chance for scar treatment. Treated areas regain characteristics similar to normal skin, becoming more elastic and softer. Moreover, this effect allows in the case of facial scars a gradual recovery of mimic, and in areas of movements an improved motility (**Figs. 1–6**).

Our clinical findings are supported by objective evidence and positive patient perception. In fact, measurements obtained with a Durometer, which is an instrument widely used to evaluate sclerodermic skin and recently used as a scar objective

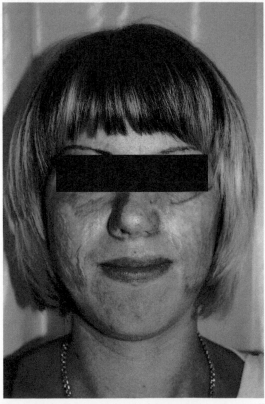

Fig. 1. Patient affected by a face burn with mimic impairment.

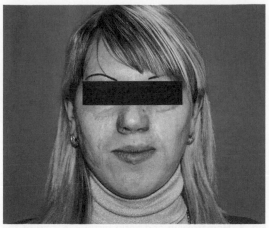

Fig. 2. Postoperative image after two autologous fat grafting procedures with local amelioration and increase in scar softness and appearance.

evaluation tool, showed a significant reduction of the area treated demonstrating scar hardness reduction after treatment.

We were able to treat cases that could not be treated with other types of surgical and nonsurgical procedures because of the high risk of suboptimal results or possible recurrence. Thus, we are persuaded that autologous fat grafting is an innovative surgical option for scar tissue treatment that provides an effective approach in cases that cannot be treated with traditional procedures.[28]

Our clinical results rely on mesenchymal stem cells and adipocyte-derived products contained

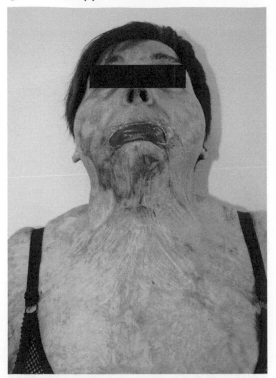

Fig. 4. Postoperative image after three autologous fat grafting procedures and skin grafting in the central area, which reveals improvement in movements and skin quality.

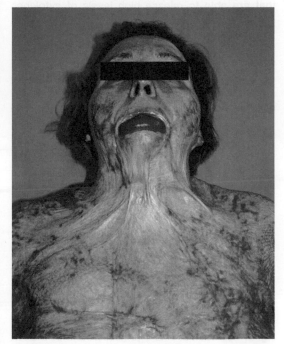

Fig. 3. Wide burn area in the neck region with important impairment to motility caused by fibrotic bridles.

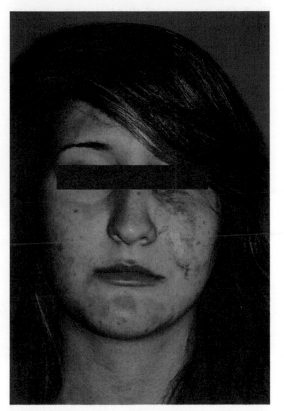

Fig. 5. Surgical scar after vascular malformation removal in the left cheek.

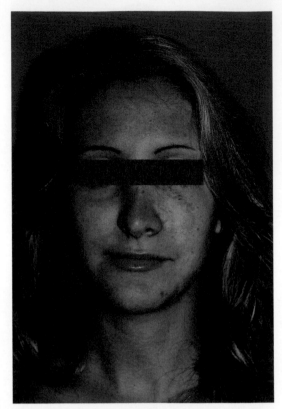

Fig. 6. Skin improvement after treatment with restoration of appearance now similar to normal skin.

in the graft, although the exact role of each component in the scar release process remains to be determined. Probably, the tissue remodeling described is created by local action of cytokines, growth factors, angiogenic factors, enzymes, and

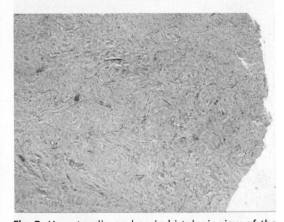

Fig. 7. Hematoxylin and eosin histologic view of the scar area before fat injection. Note the typical appearance of the scar and the cellular necrosis around the hair follicle (original magnification ×4). (*From* Coleman SR, Mazzola RF. Fat injection: from filling to regeneration. St Louis (MO): Quality Medical Publishing, Inc; 2009; with permission.)

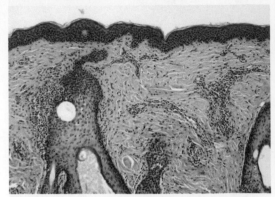

Fig. 8. Hematoxylin and eosin histologic view of the scar area 1 month after fat injection. Note the epithelial hyperplasia, dermal papillae organization, and the presence of new blood vessels (neoangiogenesis) (original magnification ×4). (*From* Coleman SR, Mazzola RF. Fat injection: from filling to regeneration. St Louis (MO): Quality Medical Publishing, Inc; 2009; with permission.)

cellular components leading to the formation of new blood vessels, achieving fibrotic tissue remodeling and a new inflammation response (**Figs. 7** and **8**). Moreover, the high content of mesenchymal and hematopoietic stem cells from this source offers the possibility of augmented tolerogenic processes by decreasing ongoing inflammation.[29]

Centrifugation concentrates cells with high clonogenic, proliferative, and differentiative abilities that are able to release high levels of cytokines and chemokines achieving a significant increase in the regenerative abilities of tissue injected.

We adopted autologous fat grafting regenerative effects also on chronic hard-to-heal wounds of small to moderate size not responding to advanced dressings, obtaining final closure after one or more procedures (**Figs. 9** and **10**). The

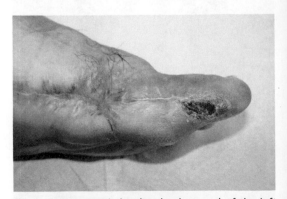

Fig. 9. Posttraumatic hard to-heal wound of the left foot already submitted to advanced dressing without showing any improvement.

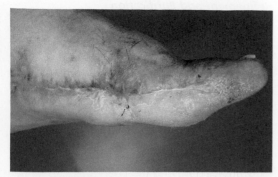

Fig. 10. Postoperative image after one procedure (3-month follow-up), which shows complete re-epithelization.

treatment stimulates re-epithelization of chronic ulcer and enhances perilesional tissue, increasing elasticity and softness, and obtaining pain control. Our experience shows the therapeutic effect of autologous fat grafting, treating both scar tissue and chronic ulcers based on its regenerative potentials.

SUPPLEMENTARY DATA

Supplementary data related to this article can be found online at http://dx.doi.org/10.1016/j.cps.2015.03.008.

REFERENCES

1. Zuk PA, Zhu M, De Ugarte DA, et al. Human adipose tissue is a source of multipotent stem cells. Mol Biol Cell 2002;13:4279–95.
2. Erickson GR, Gimble JM, Franklin DM, et al. Chondrogenic potential of adipose tissue-derived stromal cells in vitro and in vivo. Biochem Biophys Res Commun 2002;290:763–9.
3. Mizuno H, Zuk PA, Zhu M, et al. Myogenic differentiation by human processed lipoaspirate cells. Plast Reconstr Surg 2002;109:199–211.
4. Coleman SR. Long-term survival of fat transplants: controlled demonstrations. Aesthetic Plast Surg 1995;19:421–5.
5. Coleman SR. Facial augmentation with structural fat grafting. Clin Plast Surg 2006;33:567–77.
6. Rigotti G, Marchi A, Galiè M, et al. Clinical treatment of radiotherapy tissue damage by lipoaspirate transplant: a healing process mediated by adipose-derived adult stem cell. Plast Reconstr Surg 2007; 119:1409–22.
7. Klinger M, Marazzi M, Vigo D, et al. Fat injection for cases of severe burn outcomes: a new perspective of scar remodeling and reduction. Aesthetic Plast Surg 2008;32:465.
8. Klinger FM, Vinci V, Forcellini D, et al. Basic science review on adipose tissue for clinicians. Plast Reconstr Surg 2011;128:829–30.
9. Klinger M, Caviggioli F, Klinger FM, et al. Autologous fat graft in scar treatment. J Craniofac Surg 2013; 24(5):1610–5.
10. Klinger M, Caviggioli F, Klinger F, et al. Scar remodeling following burn injuries. In: Coleman SR, Mazzola RF, editors. Fat injection: from filling to regeneration. St Louis (MO): Quality Medical Publishing; 2009. p. 227–42.
11. Vinci V, Borbon G, Codolini L, et al. Fat grafting versus adipose-derived stem cell therapy: distinguishing indications, techniques, and outcomes. Aesthetic Plast Surg 2013;37(4):856–7.
12. Caviggioli F, Maione L, Vinci V, et al. The most current algorithms for the treatment and prevention of hypertrophic scars and keloids. Plast Reconstr Surg 2010;126(3):1130–1.
13. Caviggioli F, Villani F, Forcellini D, et al. Nipple resuscitation by lipostructure in burn sequelae and scar retraction. Plast Reconstr Surg 2010;125(4):174e–6e.
14. Caviggioli F, Klinger F, Villani F, et al. Correction of cicatricial ectropion by autologous fat graft. Aesthetic Plast Surg 2008;32(3):555–7.
15. Caviggioli F, Vinci V, Maione L, et al. Autologous fat grafting in secondary breast reconstruction. Ann Plast Surg 2013;70(1):119.
16. Caviggioli F, Maione L, Forcellini D, et al. Autologous fat graft in postmastectomy pain syndrome. Plast Reconstr Surg 2011;128(2):349–52.
17. Maione L, Vinci V, Caviggioli F, et al. Autologous fat graft in postmastectomy pain syndrome following breast conservative surgery and radiotherapy. Aesthetic Plast Surg 2014;38(3):528–32.
18. Gaetani P, Klinger M, Levi D, et al. Treatment of chronic headache of cervical origin with lipostructure: an observational study. Headache 2013;53(3):507–13.
19. Klinger M, Villani F, Klinger F, et al. Anatomical variations of the occipital nerves: implications for the treatment of chronic headaches. Plast Reconstr Surg 2009;124:1727–8.
20. Lisa A, Maione L, Vinci V, et al. A systematic review of peripheral nerve interventional treatments for chronic headaches. Ann Plast Surg 2014;72(4): 439–45.
21. Caviggioli F, Giannasi S, Vinci V, et al. Five-year outcome of surgical treatment of migraine headaches. Plast Reconstr Surg 2011;128(5):564e–5e [author reply: 565e].
22. Caviggioli F, Giannasi S, Vinci V, et al. Neurovascular compression of the greater occipital nerve: implications for migraine headaches. Plast Reconstr Surg 2012;129(2):353e–4e.
23. Klinger M, Caviggioli F, Vinci V, et al. Treatment of chronic post-traumatic ulcers using autologous fat graft. Plast Reconstr Surg 2010;126:154e–5e.

24. Klinger FM, Caviggioli F, Forcellini D, et al. Breast fistula repair after autologous fat graft: a case report. Case Rep Med 2011;2011:547387.

25. Ibatici A, Caviggioli F, Valeriano V, et al. Comparison of cell number, viability, phenotypic profile, clonogenic, and proliferative potential of adipose-derived stem cell populations between centrifuged and noncentrifuged fat. Aesthetic Plast Surg 2014;38(5):985–93.

26. Caviggioli F, Forcellini D, Vinci V, et al. Employment of needles: a different technique for fat placement. Plast Reconstr Surg 2012;130(2):373e–4e.

27. Maione L, Vinci V, Klinger M, et al. Autologous fat graft by needle: analysis of complications after 1000 patients. Ann Plast Surg 2015;74(3): 277–80.

28. Del Papa N, Caviggioli F, Sambataro D, et al. Autologous fat grafting in the treatment of fibrotic perioral changes in patients with systemic sclerosis. Cell Transplant 2015;24(1):63–72.

29. Ichim TE, Harman RJ, Min WP, et al. Autologous stromal vascular fraction cells: a tool for facilitating tolerance in rheumatic disease. Cell Immunol 2010;264(1):7–17.

Regenerative Approach to Scleroderma with Fat Grafting

Guy Magalon, MD[a,b,*], Aurélie Daumas, MD[c],
Nolwenn Sautereau, MD[c], Jérémy Magalon, PharmD[b],
Florence Sabatier, PharmD, PhD[b,d], Brigitte Granel, MD[c,d]

KEYWORDS

- Systemic sclerosis • Cell therapy • Microfat injection • Stromal vascular fraction • Fat grafting
- Autologous fat graft • Adipose tissue

KEY POINTS

- Systemic sclerosis (SSc) is a rare autoimmune disease characterized by skin fibrosis, microvascular damage, and organ dysfunction.
- Facial manifestations in SSc are disfiguring and lead to social disability with psychological distress.
- Hand involvement in SSc can lead to a severe disability, with no effective therapy.
- Adipose-tissue-derived stem cell therapy has emerged as a therapeutic alternative for regeneration and repair of damaged tissues.
- Patients with SSc can benefit from fat grafting: microfat injection in the face to improve skin pliability and quality with esthetic benefit, and injection of the autologous adipose-tissue-derived stromal vascular fraction (ADSVF) in fingers for a trophic effect.

Three surgical technique videos accompany this article showing the authors approach to the treatment of the face and of the hands in systemic sclerosis patients, and the inside of 2-mm, 14-gauge cannula harvesting and microfat injection with 0.8-mm, 21-gauge cannula at http://www.plasticsurgery.theclinics.com/

INTRODUCTION

SSc (scleroderma) is a chronic systemic autoimmune disease characterized by microvascular abnormalities and progressive skin and internal organ fibrosis.[1] Life-threatening organ lesions leading to pulmonary arterial hypertension, pulmonary fibrosis, and scleroderma renal crisis only affect a minority of patients. By contrast, lesions of the hands and face are almost always present. Although not life-threatening, these manifestations are very obvious, hard to conceal, and lead to disability and worsening quality of life.[2–4] Facial symptoms are associated with cosmetic

Author disclosure: G. Magalon has the following potential conflicts of interest to report: consultant for the Thiebaud Medical Device; financial grants and other support for research and honorarium as consultant.
[a] Plastic Surgery Department, Assistance Publique Hôpitaux de Marseilles (AP-HM), Aix-Marseilles University, 13005 Marseilles, France; [b] Culture and Cell Therapy Laboratory, INSERM CBT-1409, Assistance Publique Hôpitaux de Marseilles (AP-HM), Aix-Marseilles University, 13005 Marseilles, France; [c] Internal Medicine Department, Assistance Publique Hôpitaux de Marseilles (AP-HM), Aix-Marseilles University, 13010 Marseilles, France; [d] Vascular Research Center Marseilles, INSERM UMRS-1076, Aix-Marseilles University, 13005 Marseilles, France
* Corresponding author. Conception Hospital, Assistance Publique Hôpitaux de Marseilles (AP-HM), 13005 Marseilles, France.
E-mail address: secretariat.magalon@gmail.com

Clin Plastic Surg 42 (2015) 353–364
http://dx.doi.org/10.1016/j.cps.2015.03.009
0094-1298/15/$ – see front matter © 2015 Elsevier Inc. All rights reserved.

plasticsurgery.theclinics.com

disfigurement and limited expression with mask-like stiffness of the face. Lesions in the hand lead to substantial difficulty in performing everyday tasks (such as dressing, eating, and applying makeup) as well as an increased risk of chronic digital ulcers (DUs). Therapeutic interventions in this disease are mainly based on the use of vasodilators. No antifibrotic treatment has proven effective. Unlike other autoimmune diseases, immunosuppressive drugs have a limited clinical interest.[5–10] Thus, functional improvement of hand motion and face appearance represent a real challenge for physicians and a priority for patients who often feel that this aspect of their disease is neglected.

Use of adipose tissue as filling product in plastic and esthetic surgery is an ancient technique. Significant renewal of interest in this approach for the restoration of all volume defects was observed after the description of the LipoStructure® technique by Coleman.[11–13] Recently, identification and characterization of the ADSVF, a population that includes mesenchymal-like stem cells, endothelial progenitor cells, and hematopoietic cells, have revolutionized the science showing that adipose tissue is a valuable source of cells with multipotency as well as angiogenic and immunomodulatory properties that facilitate tissue repair. The ease of harvest by liposuction and the abundance of these cells (by comparison to bone marrow) avoid the need for ex vivo expansion before clinical use. Because of these practical factors and the stromal vascular fraction's ability to differentiate and secrete immunomodulatory, angiogenic, antiapoptotic, and hematopoietic factors, use of adipose tissue is becoming more attractive and is expanding in regenerative medicine.[14–19]

In this article, the authors present their clinical approach using adipose tissue in the treatment of the face and hands of patients with SSc.

PATHOLOGY OF SCLERODERMA
Face

Involvement of the face with associated oral complications, esthetic changes, and impairment of the patient's self-image is found in over 90% of patients with SSc.[3,20,21]

Fig. 1 and **Table 1** illustrate the main orofacial findings in patients with SSc.

Several validated tools have been developed for assessing the involvement of the face. Skin involvement is usually assessed by the Rodnan skin score. This semiquantitative score rates the severity of skin sclerosis from 0 (normal) to 3 (most severe). Xerostomia can be easily measured

by sugar test (time to melt a sugar on the tongue, without crunching it) and with the xerostomia inventory index. Mouth opening is assessed in centimeters by measuring the distance between the tips of upper and lower incisive teeth. Elastosonography and three-dimensional photographs can also be used. Mouth-related disability can be assessed by the Mouth Handicap in Systemic Sclerosis (MHISS) scale, which is the first mouth-specific disability outcome measure designed for patients with SSc.[3] This scale evaluates 3 factors: reduced mouth opening, sicca syndrome, and esthetic concerns. Although mouth disability seems to have less weight than hand disability in total disability, the MHISS score explained up to 36% of the variance of the Health Assessment Questionnaire score. This fact highlights the need to specifically assess disability involving the mouth in patients with SSc. Rehabilitation and management of the face is mainly based on physiotherapy with mimic exercises, massage, and self-administered home-based exercises. Mouth and dental care are not specific.

Some case reports have shown the efficacy of autologous fat grafting in the treatment of linear scleroderma.[22,23] Besides the volumizing effect of mechanical lipofilling, autologous fat grafting also seems to produce trophic and angiogenic effects. The use of autologous grafting of adipose tissue seems to have substantial potential to correct signs of face involvement in SSc.

Hands

Involvement of the hand is common in patients with SSc and represents a large burden in work and daily activities. Hand disability has a multifactorial origin with microvascular lesions, skin sclerosis, tendon retraction, bone and articular involvement, and subcutaneous calcinosis.[4,24–31] Each of these lesions causes pain, functional impairment, esthetic issues, and psychological distress.

Vascular involvement

Vascular dysfunction including Raynaud's phenomenon (paroxysmal vasospasm) (**Fig. 2**), acrocyanosis (permanent ischemia), and subsequently DUs with their potential complications (infections, digital necrosis, autoamputation) are the main manifestations. Raynaud's phenomenon occurs in almost all (95%) patients with SSc. DUs, defined as necrotic lesions that occur either at the pulp of the digits (ischemic DUs) or over bony prominences (mechanical DUs), occur in up to 50% of patients with limited or diffuse SSc. DUs typically occur early in the course of SSc. A study assessing functional limitations owing to

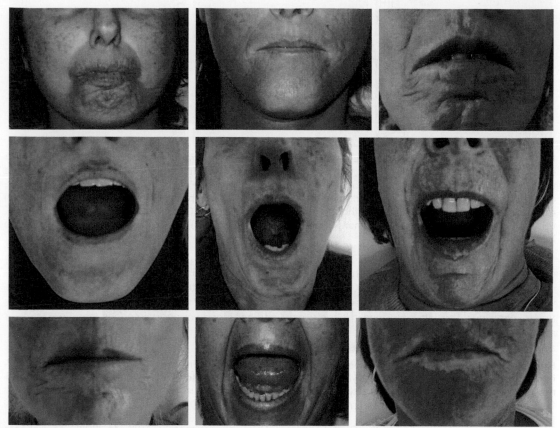

Fig. 1. Various aspects of SSc face involvement showing skin sclerosis, cutaneous wrinkles, vertical furrows that develop around the mouth, sharp nose and lip retraction, telangiectasia, hypopigmentation and hyperpigmentation, and reduction of mouth opening.

Table 1
Orofacial findings in patients with SSc

Orofacial Findings	Commentaries
Skin sclerosis of the face	Very frequent, around 90% of cases. The face becomes amimic or without expression, cutaneous wrinkles disappear, vertical furrows develop around the mouth because of retraction of the skin, the nose becomes sharp, and the lips thin
Telangiectasia	Especially located in the face, lips, or the inside of the mouth; they can lead to severe esthetic concerns
Skin pigmentation abnormalities	Hypopigmentation and hyperpigmentation mostly observed in the diffuse cutaneous form of scleroderma. Vitiligo is possible
Sicca syndrome	Sicca syndrome is detected in approximately 70% of patients with SSc. It is secondary to salivary gland fibrosis
Diminished mouth opening	Frequent, around 60%. Thinning of lips and reduction of mouth width (microcheilia) and opening (microstomia) with consequent difficult dental care
Osteolysis of mandibular angles	Mandibular bone resorption is mainly encountered in patients with marked facial skin fibrosis: chewing and swallowing movements may be impaired, pain is often reported
Altered dentition and difficulties during dental care	Oromucosal involvement include ulcerations, dry mouth, periodontitis, wide periodontal ligament space, dental root resorption, and loose teeth

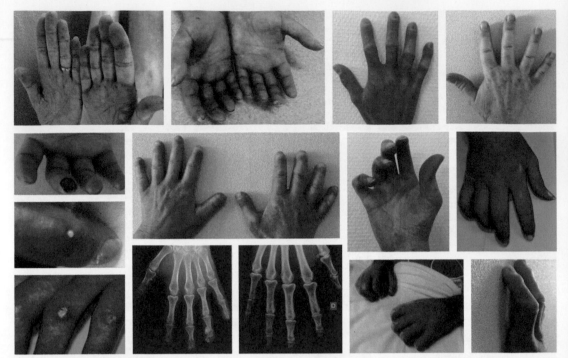

Fig. 2. Various aspects of SSc hand involvement showing acrocyanosis, palmar telangiectasia, sclerodactyly, puffing hand, tightened finger on the underlying bone, various types of DUs (ischemic, mechanic, and related to calcinosis), acro-osteolysis, and claw deformity.

DUs among patients enrolled in the Digital Ulcer Outcome (DUO) Registry showed for patients with 0, 1 to 2, and 3 or more DUs at enrollment an increasing mean overall work impairment. Similarly, the ability to perform daily activities was impaired in patients with DUs and this impairment increased with the number of DUs.

Skin involvement

Skin sclerosis is characterized by variable extent and severity of skin thickening and hardening. Edematous swelling and erythema may precede skin induration. On the hands, this condition is called sclerodactyly (see **Fig. 2**). As the disease progresses further, however, the skin loses its ability to stretch and becomes shiny because it tightens across the underlying bone. Eventually, in severe cases, the fingers may lose the ability to move, with vicious attitude leading to claw deformities (see **Fig. 2**).

Flat red marks, known as telangiectasias (see **Fig. 2**), may appear in various locations, especially in the palms. Although they can cause esthetic concerns, they do not cause functional disturbance.

Calcinosis (see **Fig. 2**) is characterized by calcium deposition in skin and subcutaneous tissues. Calcinosis is commonly associated with SSc; approximately 10% to 30% of patients develop calcinosis. These deposits are typically found on the fingers, hands, and on the skin above wrists, elbows, and knees. Calcinosis can lead to functional impairment, painful ulcers, and infections.

Bone and joint involvement

Distal phalangeal resorption with bone loss (acro-osteolysis) can be observed in SSc (see **Fig. 2**). Arthralgia and arthritis are observed in around 50% of cases. Metacarpophalangeal and proximal interphalangeal arthritis are also frequent. This joint destruction is not as severe as it is in rheumatoid arthritis but can lead to finger deformities and claw hand deformity.

Clinical measures for hand involvement evaluation include: (1) the semiquantitative estimation of skin thickness (modified Rodnan skin score applied to hands, score 0–18); (2) a visual analog scale of pain in the hands; (3) mobility and strength tests such as Kapandji test, grip and pinch strength, and measurement of the intercommissural distances; (4) the Hand Mobility in Scleroderma index, which specifically assesses hand global mobility in patients with SSc, but does not evaluate hand disability for activities of daily living; and (5) the Cochin Hand Function

Scale (CHFS), a functional disability questionnaire about daily activities validated in rheumatoid arthritis and hand osteoarthritis, as well as SSc. The CHFS is a valid instrument for assessing hand disability in patients with SSc. It was shown that hand functional disability is the major component of global disability, contributing to 75% of global disability in patients.[4]

To date, therapeutic interventions for patients with hands affected by SSc have mainly focused on the treatment of vascular manifestations such as Raynaud's phenomenon and DUs. Patients can get some relief with physiotherapy. Unfortunately, there is scant research showing that exercise stops the worsening of scleroderma (Videos 1 and 2). Full rehabilitation is rarely guaranteed, but function can be retained through physiotherapy. Movement can help retard the contractures and help the patient maintain strength and range of motion.[5–10]

ADIPOSE-TISSUE-BASED THERAPY IN SYSTEMIC SCLEROSIS

Over the past few years, stem cell therapy has emerged as a novel therapeutic approach for various diseases including ischemic diseases, wound repair, and tissue regeneration.[14–19,32] The adipose tissue contains various cells such as adipose-derived stem/stromal cells, endothelial progenitor cells, and immune cells, which act together for tissue repair and regeneration. The abundant supply of fat tissue, the ease of isolation, the ability to secrete angiogenic growth factors, and the abundance of stem/progenitor cells make adipose-based therapy ideal for ischemic and nonhealing wounds. In this disease, adipose-derived cell therapy seems to be an attractive source and worthy of attention for clinical translation.

TREATMENT OF THE FACE

Reinjection of autologous fat tissue has volumizing and trophic properties. This technique has been codified by Coleman.[11,12] However, the special context of SSc requires certain modifications to this approach, in particular, harvesting and implanting smaller morsels or packets of adipose tissue.[33] Thus, microreinjection is an evolution of the art. The tissue is aspirated by a 2-mm (14-gauge) cannula, with openings of less than 1-mm, which harvests fat lobules of about 600-µm. Tissue is reimplanted using a 0.8-mm (21-gauge) placement cannula. This minimally invasive technique is used to treat the face of the patient with scleroderma.

Surgical Technique

During the first consultation (after a clinical and photographic analysis), the surgeon defines the amount of adipose tissue necessary and the areas from which this tissue can be harvested (**Fig. 3**). Preferred harvesting areas include the abdomen, hips, and inner side of the knees; the most preferred location for small quantities is the inner side of the knees. The entire procedure takes place under local anesthesia (supplemented with conscious sedation if needed) and can be performed either as an outpatient or in inpatient care.

Sampling and infiltration

The first step is anesthesia of the entry point with a 3-mL syringe and a 30-gauge needle. An incision is then made with a 14-gauge needle, before inserting the infiltration cannula of the same diameter (14-gauge, 2-mm). For infiltration, the authors use a modified Klein solution containing 800 mg lidocaine and adrenaline 1/1,000,000 with a wet technique. Aspiration is performed using a 10-mL syringe with less than 1-mL vacuum.

Purification

Two techniques can be used for purification of the product:

- The standard for fat graft processing has long been centrifugation. For microfat, the authors recommend centrifugation for 1 or 2 minutes at 1200 g. The lower phase containing the infiltration liquid is removed. In the authors' experience, there is minimal oil from disrupted fat.
- Filtration using the PureGraft™ (Cytori Therapeutics, Inc, San Diego, CA, USA) closed membrane filtration system can be used as an alternative. Tumescent fluid, blood cells, debris, and oil are removed by this system leaving filtered living purified fat.

With both techniques, the pure fatty tissue is transferred via a Luer Lock connector from the 10-mL syringe into multiple 1-mL syringes for implantation. In order to prevent air bubbles, the connector is first placed on the 10-mL syringe and primed with tissue before connecting to the 1-mL syringe.

Placement/implantation

The entry points are anesthetized. The skin barrier is crossed with a 21-gauge needle or 0.8-mm cannula in the same direction In which the minicannula (21-gauge, 0.8-mm) needs to be introduced. Tissue may be injected in all areas, but especially in the superficial plane, as close to the skin level as can be achieved without risk of irregularities. The tissue can be implanted in several planes in

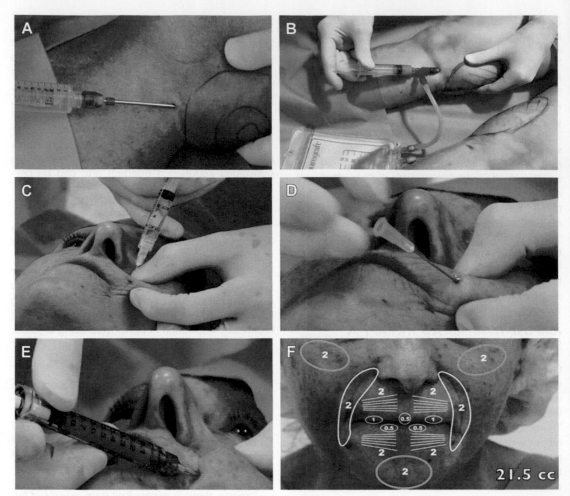

Fig. 3. Surgical technique using microfat in the treatment of the face. (*A*) Local infiltration in the inner part of the knee. (*B*) Microharvesting with a closed system. (*C*) Local anesthesia of the face. (*D*) Entry point with a 21-gauge needle (0.8-mm). (*E*). Fat injection with a 1-mL syringe and 21-gauge (0.8-mm) cannula. (*F*) Fat placement and quantities.

different directions knowing that micrografts are on the order of 500-μm and contain only a few hundred cells.

Postoperative period

The postoperative course is extremely simple. There are no painful symptoms, the swelling is extremely small, and there is normally little bruising. The result is stable after the second post-operative month. An improvement in the quality of skin, esthetic appearance, face pain, and mouth opening can be observed at 6 months.

Case 1 A 57-year-old woman with SSc consulted for functional and cosmetic improvement of her face. SSc was diagnosed in 2006 and was characterized by skin sclerosis above her forearm (diffuse cutaneous form of the disease), Raynaud's

phenomenon complicated by ischemic DUs, poly-arthritis, upper digestive tract symptoms with typical pattern of esophagus involvement at manometry, and sicca syndrome. Alteration of alveolar diffusion on pulmonary function test was observed, without a restrictive pattern. She did not have pulmonary arterial hypertension or renal crisis. She was taking low-dose steroids, metho-trexate, folic acid, nifedipine, bosentan, and eso-meprazole and applying emollient creams on her face twice a day. Her medical history did not include any other disease, alcohol, or smoking. Biological investigations showed positive results for anticentromere antibodies, with normal results of blood tests as well as renal and liver function tests and no deficiency of iron or vitamins B_{12} and B_9. Her physical examination revealed marked skin thickening on the face with a Rodnan skin score applied to face at 2/3. At entry, the MHISS score was at 36/48, the Xerostomia Inventory Index was at 52/55, sugar test was at 4 minutes, 42 seconds, and mouth opening was at 25-mm. According to the surgical procedure described above, lipoaspiration of 50-mL of fat from the inner part of the knees was performed and the Pure-Graft™ filtration device was used. In the same operating time, 19.8-mL of microfat was reinjected around the lips. No specific medication was given after the treatment except for mild analgesics. Tolerance was good, and when asked 6 months later, the patient was very satisfied with all the following parameters showing improvement in comparison to baseline: MHISS score was at 23/48, Xerostomia Inventory Index was at 44/55, sugar test was at 2 minutes, 54 seconds, and mouth opening was at 35-mm. **Fig. 4** demonstrates a representative example.

TREATMENT OF THE HAND

The treatment for hands is performed using a cell therapy protocol, which uses ADSVF (Video 3). Because of skin fibrosis, microfat injection is unthinkable in the hands owing to the risk of ischemia related to the volume effect.[34] ADSVF is prepared using the Celution® System (Cytori Therapeutics, Inc).

Surgical Technique

In the operating room, adipose tissue collection and ADSVF injection are conducted under conscious sedation; harvesting areas are anesthetized (**Fig. 5**).

Sampling and infiltration

The entry points are anesthetized with a 3-mL syringe and a 30-gauge needle. For infiltration, the authors use a modified Klein solution containing 800 mg lidocaine and adrenaline 1/1,000,000 with the wet technique. After making the guidance hole with a 14-gauge needle, infiltration is performed with a 2-mm cannula in the knees, abdomen, and hips and, if necessary, in the back. For collection, the authors use a Khouri cannula with 12 holes 2.5-mm long × 1.5-mm wide or a standard Coleman harvesting cannula. Harvesting is performed with a 10-mL syringe in a closed circuit with 2 terminal 4 × 2-mm openings with a 2-way nonreturn adipose tissue valve, sterile tubing, and a 250-mL collection bag. Tissue is collected using low vacuum. When the bag is filled, it is placed in a sterile double pack and transported to the cell therapy laboratory.

Purification

Once harvesting is complete, the bag is immediately transported to the registered cell therapy unit. ADSVF is obtained within 2 h after lipoaspiration using the automated processing Celution800/CRS system (Cytori Therapeutics, Inc). Fat tissue is processed in the Celution® System according to the manufacturer's instructions. Briefly, tissue is transferred into the canister, washed, and rinsed with Ringer lactate at 37°C after which the processing enzyme is prepared and injected. Upon completion of digestion, the system automatically washes and concentrates the ADSVF cells. After the centrifugation step, 2.5-mL of ADSVF is collected from each side to make up a total of 5-mL. This sample is then diluted into 11-mL of Ringer lactate and then transferred in 10 doses (1-mL), one for each finger. The remaining volume is used for sterility testing and biological characterization. Total viable nucleated cell recovery and viability percentage are determined using the NucleoCounter® NC-100™ (ChemoMetec, Denmark). Cellular components are identified by flow cytometry using a Beckman Navios instrument (Beckman Coulter, Miami, FL, USA) with a

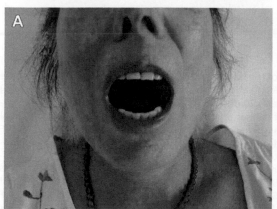
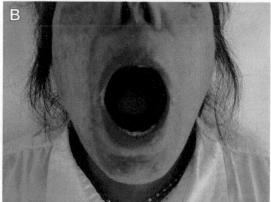

Fig. 4. Mouth opening before (A) and 6 months after (B) microfat injection.

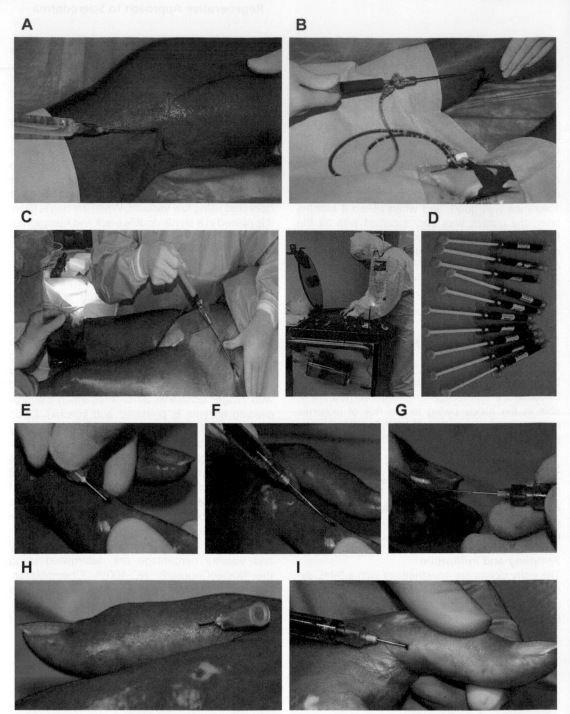

Fig. 5. Surgical technique using ADSVF in the treatment of the hands. (*A*) Local infiltration in the inner part of the knee. (*B*) Microharvesting with a closed system in the knee. (*C*) Microharvesting with a closed system in the hip. (*D*) ADSVF extraction with the Celution® System and obtaining 10 doses (1 for each finger) of diluted ADSVF. (*E*) Injection orifice for long fingers is located at the union of palmar and dorsal surfaces at the level of the proximal interphalangeal joints. Entry is performed using a 25-gauge needle (0.5-mm). (*F*) Injection of 0.25-mL of ADSVF using a 25-gauge (0.5-mm) reinforced cannula placed into the subcutaneous tissue in contact with the neurovascular pedicles using a retrotracing technique from distal to proximal. (*G*) Injection of 0.25-mL of ADSVF using a 25-gauge (0.5-mm) reinforced cannula placed into the subcutaneous tissue in contact with the neurovascular pedicles using a retrotracing technique from proximal to distal. (*H*) Injection orifice for the thumb is located at the level of metacarpophalangeal joint. Entry is performed using a 25-gauge needle (0.5-mm). (*I*) Injection of 0.5-mL of ADSVF into each lateral side of the thumb using a 25-gauge (0.5-mm) reinforced cannula placed into the subcutaneous tissue in contact with the neurovascular pedicles using a retrotracing technique from distal to proximal.

panel of cell surface makers in agreement with International Federation for Adipose Therapeutics and Science and the International Society for Cellular Therapy recommendations. The markers CD45, CD34, CD90, CD146, and CD14 are used in combination with deep red fluorescing anthraquinone (DRAQ5) and diamidinophenylindole (DAPI) to exclude debris, red blood cells, and dead cells. The frequency of adipose-derived mesenchymal-like stem cells is estimated using the colony-forming unit-fibroblast (CFU-F) clonogenic assay.

Placement

The ADSVF cells are transported in a controlled manner to the operating room. The injection points are marked on the edges of each finger, at the junction of palmar and dorsal faces. Entry is performed using a 25-gauge needle (0.5-mm). ADSVF cells are then injected using a 25-gauge (0.5-mm) reinforced cannula placed into the subcutaneous tissue in contact with the neurovascular pedicles: 0.5-mL of the solution is injected into lateral side of each digit, using a retrotracing technique, from distal to proximal. Entry points are positioned at the metacarpophalangeal joint for the thumb, and the proximal interphalangeal joint where the palmar and dorsal skin joins for long fingers. The operation is continued on all fingers of the first hand before proceeding with the same injections on the other hand. Both hands are treated over a period of approximately 20 minutes.

In order to have maximal visibility when introducing the cannula, it is essential that a magnifying glass be used. As the patient has received neuroleptanalgesia, the postsurgical recovery is simple.

Postoperative period

Patients are discharge from the hospital a few hours after surgery. No dressing is required. Resumption of normal activities is possible immediately. Abdominal lipoaspiration sample points heal rapidly, and the points of entry for ADSVF injection heal as soon as the next day. Abdominal bruises and pain induced by the lipoaspiration can be observed, but these symptoms spontaneously disappear within a few days.

Case 1 A 34-year old woman with SSc consulted for therapeutic advice. SSc was recently diagnosed based on the following criteria: rapidly progressive skin sclerosis (diffuse cutaneous form of the disease), Raynaud's phenomenon complicated by ischemic DUs, acrocyanosis and severe sclerodactyly, and upper digestive tract symptoms with typical pattern of esophagus involvement at manometry. Thoracic computed tomography revealed mild fibrosis with alteration

of alveolar diffusion on pulmonary function test, without a restrictive pattern. She did not have pulmonary arterial hypertension or renal crisis. Biological investigations gave positive results for antitopoisomerase I antibodies, with normal results of blood tests as well as renal and liver function tests. She was taking lercanidipine and esomeprazole. She had been treated with intravenous iloprost without efficacy. Her medical history did not include any other disease, alcohol, or smoking. She was a dental prosthetist and stopped working because of disability of hands.

Her physical examination revealed marked skin thickening with a global Rodnan skin score of 32, acrocyanosis, sclerodactyly, and an ischemic DU on the pad of the third finger of the left hand. According to the surgical procedure described above, lipoaspiration of 165-mL of abdominal fat was performed and ADSVF was isolated with the Celution® System to be reinjected into her fingers. No specific medication was given after the treatment except for mild analgesics. Tolerance was good, and when asked 6 months later, the patient declared to be satisfied with all the following parameters showing improvement in comparison to baseline: decrease in Raynaud phenomenon's severity from 6/10 to 2/10 (Raynaud Condition Score), decrease in CHFS from 51/90 to 34/90, regression of the DU, decrease of mean circumference of the fingers, decrease in Rodnan skin score applied to hand from 18 to 15, and improvement in quality of life.

Fig. 6 demonstrates a representative example.

DISCUSSION

The authors carried out an open-label, single-arm, monocentric trial with 6-month follow-up among 12 female patients with SSc with CHFS greater than 20/90.[34] No severe adverse events occurred during the procedure and follow-up. Four minor adverse events reported by 4 patients were potentially related to the procedure: 2 abdominal bruises induced by the lipoaspiration of 7 and 15 days duration, 1 transient paresthesia on the lateral side of the left fifth finger persisting for 11 days postsurgery, and 1 pain located on the lateral side of the left thumb persisting for 13 days postsurgery. These events spontaneously resolved. Abdominal lipoaspiration sample points healed in less than 7 days postsurgery, and the points of entry for ADSVF injection healed as soon as the next day. Abdominal pain remained moderate and transient. A significant improvement in hand disability and pain, Raynaud's phenomenon, finger edema, and quality of life was observed. This study outlines the safety of the autologous ADSVF cell

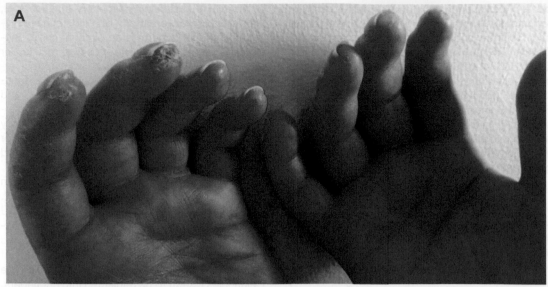

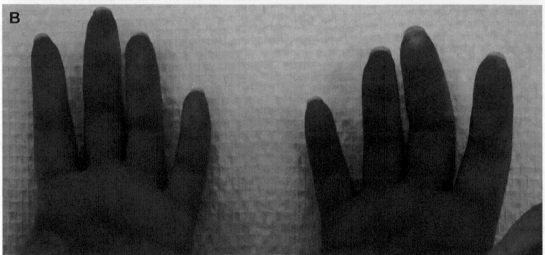

Fig. 6. Fingers before (A) and 6 months after (B) ADSVF injection.

injection in the hands of patients with SSc with encouraging results with regard to efficacy at 6 months with persistent effect at 12 months. Confirmation in a randomized placebo-controlled trial on a larger population of patients is required.

ADSVF therapy for the hands of patients with SSc is mainly indicated when hand disability is moderate to severe and persistent despite optimal medications, such as oral calcium channel blockers, endothelin 1 receptor antagonists, and phosphodiesterase 5 inhibitors, and regular physiotherapy. Patients with severe internal organ involvement, patients with finger infection, and patients with general anesthesia contraindication or taking antiplatelet agent or anticoagulant should be excluded. In the series of 12 patients with SSc, the benefit of ADSVF therapy was mainly

observed on vascular manifestations, particularly of Raynaud's phenomenon severity, DUs outcome, and hand pain, the last of these being in major part related to chronic vasospasm and DUs. The decrease of finger circumference was probably related to an improvement of finger skin edema. All together, these effects could explain the positive benefit the authors observed in hand disability and pain. These observations also suggest that ADSVF may improve vasomotor tone and microvascular perfusion. Consistently, one of the main properties of ADSVF is to promote vascular repair and angiogenesis, as documented in various experimental models of tissue ischemia.[17,35] No significant correlation was observed in the authors' study between the characteristics of the injected ADSVF (number of viable cells, proportion of the different subpopulations defined using flow cytometry, and CFU-F clonogenic test) and clinical outcomes (CHFS, hand pain, Raynaud phenomenon's severity, and quality of life). Further study in a larger cohort of patients will help delineate the phenotype of patients who best respond with this cell-based therapy.

Some limitations of this therapy are (1) a low body mass index preventing the aspiration of large quantity of fat, (2) severe and irreducible finger retractions, and (3) the need to isolate the ADSVF in an experimented cell therapy laboratory.

Concerning future perspectives, it will be interesting to evaluate the combination of fat grafting with ADSVF to have both filling and trophic effect for indications in which both these effects are wanted. By combining the lipostructure technique with the regenerative cell therapy tissue, graft longevity and positive effect could be enhanced. In SSc, applications could concern both hands and face: for hands, the association of both ischemic manifestations and mechanic ulcers related to skin tightening on bone relief, and for face, optimization of the regenerative effect of autologous fat grafting. Another perspective relies on the use of platelet-rich plasma combined with fat to ensure better survival of the grafted fat.

SUMMARY

Microfat injection in the face of patients with SSc is a safe and reliable procedure increasing facial volume and improving the quality of the skin and mouth opening. Implantation of autologous freshly isolated ADSVF population into the fingers of patients with SSc has a good safety profile with encouraging secondary efficacy end points.

ACKNOWLEDGMENTS

We thank the French Scleroderma Research Group (GFRS) for financial support given for the phase I clinical trial on safety and potential of autologous adipose-derived stromal vascular fraction in the fingers of patients with SSc.

SUPPLEMENTARY DATA

Supplementary data related to this article can be found online at http://dx.doi.org/10.1016/j.cps.2015.03.009.

REFERENCES

1. Servettaz A, Agard C, Tamby MC, et al. Systemic sclerosis: pathophysiology of a multifaceted disease. Presse Med 2006;35:1903–15.

2. Maddali Bongi S, Del Rosso A, Mikhaylova S, et al. Impact of hand face disabilities on global disability and quality of life in systemic sclerosis patients. Clin Exp Rheumatol 2014;32:S15–20.

3. Mouthon L, Rannou F, Bérezné A, et al. Development and validation of a scale for mouth handicap in systemic sclerosis: the mouth handicap in systemic sclerosis scale. Ann Rheum Dis 2007;66:1651–5.

4. Rannou F, Poiraudeau S, Berezné A, et al. Assessing disability and quality of life in systemic sclerosis: construct validities of the Cochin Hand Function Scale, Health Assessment Questionnaire (HAQ), Systemic Sclerosis HAQ, and Medical Outcomes Study 36-Item Short Form Health Survey. Arthritis Rheum 2007;57:94–102.

5. Kowal-Bielecka O, Landewé R, Avouac J, et al. EULAR recommendations for the treatment of systemic sclerosis: a report from the EULAR Scleroderma Trials and Research group (EUSTAR). Ann Rheum Dis 2009;68:620–8.

6. Korn JH, Mayes M, Matucci Cerinic M, et al. Digital ulcers in systemic sclerosis: prevention by treatment with bosentan, an oral endothelin receptor antagonist. Arthritis Rheum 2004;50:3985–93.

7. Matucci-Cerinic M, Denton CP, Furst DE, et al. Bosentan treatment of digital ulcers related to systemic sclerosis: results from the RAPIDS-2 randomised, double-blind, placebo-controlled trial. Ann Rheum Dis 2011;70:32–8.

8. Brueckner CS, Becker MO, Kroencke T, et al. Effect of sildenafil on digital ulcers in systemic sclerosis: analysis from a single centre pilot study. Ann Rheum Dis 2010;69:1475–8.

9. Wigley FM, Seibold JR, Wise RA, et al. Intravenous iloprost treatment of Raynaud's phenomenon and ischemic ulcers secondary to systemic sclerosis. J Rheumatol 1992;19:1407–14.

10. Pope JE, Bellamy N, Seibold JR, et al. A randomized, controlled trial of methotrexate versus placebo in early diffuse scleroderma. Arthritis Rheum 2001;44:1351–8.

11. Coleman SR. Long-term survival of fat transplants: controlled demonstrations. Aesthetic Plast Surg 1995;19:421–5.

12. Coleman SR. Structural fat grafting: more than a permanent filler. Plast Reconstr Surg 2006;118:108S–20S.

13. Gimble JM, Katz AJ, Bunnell BA. Adipose-derived stem cells for regenerative medicine. Circ Res 2007;100:1249–60.

14. Zuk PA, Zhu M, Ashjian P, et al. Human adipose tissue is a source of multipotent stem cells. Mol Diol Cell 2002;13:4279–95.

15. Kapur SK, Katz AJ. Review of the adipose derived stem cell secretome. Biochimie 2013;95:2222–8.

16. Leto Barone AA, Khalifian S, Lee WP, et al. Immunomodulatory effects of adipose-derived stem cells: fact or fiction? Biomed Res Int 2013;2013:383685.

17. Rehman J, Traktuev D, Li J, et al. Secretion of angio-genic and antiapoptotic factors by human adipose stromal cells. Circulation 2004;109:1292–8.

18. Lin K, Matsubara Y, Masuda Y, et al. Character-ization of adipose tissue-derived cells isolated with the Celution system. Cytotherapy 2008;10:417–26.

19. Scuderi N, Ceccarelli S, Onesti MG, et al. Human adipose-derived stromal cells for cell-based thera-pies in the treatment of systemic sclerosis. Cell Transplant 2013;22:779–95.

20. Wood RE, Lee P. Analysis of the oral manifestations of systemic sclerosis (scleroderma). Oral Surg Oral Med Oral Pathol 1988;65:172–8.

21. Vincent C, Agard C, Barbarot S, et al. Orofacial manifestations of systemic sclerosis: a study of 30 consecutive patients. Rev Med Interne 2009;30:5–11.

22. Oh CK, Lee J, Jang BS, et al. Treatment of atrophies secondary to trilinear scleroderma en coup de sabre by autologous tissue cocktail injection. Dermatol Surg 2003;29:1073–5.

23. Consorti G, Tieghi R, Clauser LC. Frontal linear scleroderma: long-term result in volumetric restora-tion of the fronto-orbital area by structural fat graft-ing. J Craniofac Surg 2012;23:263–5.

24. Mouthon L. Hand involvement in systemic sclerosis. Presse Med 2013;42:1616–26.

25. Guillevin L, Hunsche E, Denton CP, et al, DUO Registry Group. Functional impairment of systemic scleroderma patients with digital ulcerations: re-sults from the DUO Registry. Clin Exp Rheumatol 2013;31:71–80.

26. Hachulla E, Clerson P, Launay D, et al. Natural his-tory of ischemic digital ulcers in systemic sclerosis: single-center retrospective longitudinal study. J Rheumatol 2007;34:2423–30.

27. Mouthon L, Carpentier PH, Lok C, et al, ECLIPSE Study Investigators. Ischemic digital ulcers affect hand disability and pain in systemic sclerosis. J Rheumatol 2014;41:1317–23.

28. Van den Hoogen F, Khanna D, Fransen J, et al. 2013 Classification criteria for systemic sclerosis: an American College of Rheumatology/European League against Rheumatism collaborative initiative. Arthritis Rheum 2013;65:2737–47.

29. Clements PJ, Lachenbruch PA, Seibold JR, et al. Skin thickness score in systemic sclerosis: an assessment of interobserver variability in 3 indepen-dent studies. J Rheumatol 1993;20:1892–6.

30. Daumas A, Rossi P, Ariey-Bonnet D, et al. General-ized calcinosis in systemic sclerosis. QJM 2014;107:219–21.

31. Daumas A, Grob A, Faucher B, et al. Unusual cause of neck pain in systemic sclerosis. Rev Med Interne 2013;34:719–20.

32. Daumas A, Eraud J, Hautier A, et al. Interests and potentials of adipose tissue in scleroderma. Rev Med Interne 2013;34:763–9.

33. Nguyen PS, Desouches C, Gay AM, et al. Develop-ment of micro-injection as an innovative autologous fat graft technique: the use of adipose tissue as dermal filler. J Plast Reconstr Aesthet Surg 2012;65:1692–9.

34. Granel B, Daumas A, Jouve E, et al. Safety, tolera-bility and potential efficacy of injection of autologous adipose-derived stromal vascular fraction in the fin-gers of patients with systemic sclerosis: an open-label phase I trial. Ann Rheum Dis 2014. [Epub ahead of print].

35. Nakagami H, Maeda K, Morishita R, et al. Novel autologous cell therapy in ischemic limb disease through growth factor secretion by cultured adipose tissue-derived stromal cells. Arterioscler Thromb Vasc Biol 2005;25:2542–7.

Regenerative Approach to Velopharyngeal Incompetence with Fat Grafting

Riccardo F. Mazzola, MD[a],*, Giovanna Cantarella, MD[b],
Isabella C. Mazzola, MD[b]

KEYWORDS

- Velopharyngeal incompetence • Hypernasality • Nasal air escape • Nasoendoscopy • Fat grafting
- Regenerative medicine • Submucous cleft

KEY POINTS

- Mild to moderate velopharyngeal incompetence (VPI) constitutes a dilemma for surgeons. Standard techniques such as velopharyngoplasties are invasive and carry the risk of airway obstruction. Autologous fat injection offers the advantage of considerably less morbidity.
- Fat grafting to the nasopharynx should be performed under direct vision with the assistance of a rigid endoscope connected to a video system to visualize the correct injection sites.
- The level of placement is important. Fat should be introduced into the muscular layer to avoid the risk of caudal displacement, along the natural cleavage plane in the prevertebral space.
- It is mandatory to use blunt cannulas only, never sharp needles, to prevent the risk of injecting into the vessels or injury to the internal carotid artery.
- Fat grafting to the velopharyngeal port can successfully treat cases of moderate VPI while preserving the pharyngeal anatomy.

 Videonasoendoscopy pre-operative and post-operative of fat injection in a patient affected by velopharyngeal insufficiency accompanies this article at http://www. plasticsurgery.theclinics.com/

INTRODUCTION

The muscular activity of the velum and the pharyngeal walls regulates speech resonance and contributes to speech articulation. During phonation, the levator veli palatini muscle elevates the velum in an upward and backward direction while the palatopharyngeus and the pharyngeal constrictor muscles approximate the pharyngeal walls toward the midline. By this mechanism, the lateral and posterior walls of the pharynx are pulled in and the aperture between the nose and oropharynx gradually closes.

If for differing anatomy, either congenital or acquired, closure of the velopharyngeal (VP) port does not take place, the air escapes from the oropharynx into the nose, impairing normal speech articulation and resonance. This condition is termed velopharyngeal incompetence (VPI) and the ensuing resonance alteration is known as hypernasality. VPI may also affect suction and deglutition, with possible nasal regurgitation of fluids and foods.

Beginning from the second half of the nineteenth century, numerous surgical techniques have been proposed over the years to treat VPI by reducing

The authors have no disclosures.
[a] Department of Clinical Sciences and Community Health, Fondazione Ospedale Maggiore Policlinico, Ca' Granda, IRCCS, via Marchiondi 7, Milano 20122, Italy; [b] Department of Otolaryngology, Fondazione Ospedale Maggiore Policlinico, Ca' Granda, IRCCS, via Francesco Sforza 35, Milano 20122, Italy
* Corresponding author.
E-mail address: Riccardo.mazzola@fastwebnet.it

the passage between the oropharynx and naso-pharynx.[1] Such methods include: soft palate re-repair, when musculature has not been reap-proximated during primary closure or when scar tissue is present along the midline impairing palatal elevation[2]; double-opposing Z-plasty, to recreate the levator muscle sling and elongate the velum simultaneously[3]; pushback procedures, designed to lengthen the soft palate, preserving its dynamics, by moving the entire palatal fibro-mucosa backward with reduction of the space between the velum and the posterior pharyngeal wall[4]; velopharyngoplasties; and advancement of the posterior pharyngeal wall.

Velopharyngoplasties encompass the superiorly based and the less used inferiorly based pharyn-geal flap,[5–8] or the transposition of the posterior pharyngeal pillars, containing the palatopharyng-eus muscle.[9] These plasties are effective in dimin-ishing the passage between the nasal cavity and the oropharynx for management of severe VPI, but may have a relevant morbidity either in the im-mediate postoperative period, such as severe pain and risk of bleeding, or over the long term, such as snoring and obstructive sleep apnea (OSA). How-ever, they are considered an overtreatment in the presence of moderate VPI.

Advancement of the posterior pharyngeal wall is a well-known method in use since the beginning of the twentieth century.[10] A large variety of implants[11–17] or autologous tissue[18,19] have been placed over the years into the retropharyngeal space, with the aim of pushing the posterior wall of the pharynx forward to meet the velum and reduce the size of the nasopharyngeal port. To be efficacious, the implant should be located high in the pharynx at the point of the velar con-tact. Over time, however, extrusion or dislocation of the implant in a lower position along the poste-rior pharyngeal wall has often been reported, making the rationale of this technique questionable.

Recently, autologous fat transplantation to the velopharynx has been proved to be successful in the treatment of VPI.[20–25]

PATIENT SELECTION AND TREATMENT GOALS

The aims of this article are to highlight patient selection criteria for fat grafting and illustrate the technical details for making the procedure effec-tive in reducing the VP gap.

Patient selection constitutes a critical step. Fat grafting, in fact, can successfully correct only mild to moderate gaps of VP closure.

Preoperative assessment is based on a thorough evaluation performed by the surgeon together with a specially trained phoniatrician and a speech therapist.

Treatment protocol includes:

- Perceptual evaluation, with spontaneous speech and repetition of sentences and pho-nemes, designed to assess resonance, audible air escape and turbulence, articulation defects, and potential dysphonia
- Acoustic measurements, such as nasometry
- Aerodynamic evaluation to quantify the nasal air leakage
- Videofluoroscopic study of the VP port in multiple projections
- Videonasopharyngoscopy

In the authors' clinical practice, perceptual eval-uation and videonasopharyngoscopy are consid-ered the standard for patient selection, while aerodynamic measurements are performed in selected cases and for research purposes. Perceptual assessment includes video recording of several speech samples using a professional microphone. The videos are blindly evaluated by independent listeners with specific expertise in VP function. The information gained from such studies provides us with quantifiable data and as-sists us to critically and blindly evaluate our re-sults. It is of critical importance to distinguish between VP incompetence and VP dysfunction that can be treated conservatively by speech ther-apy without the need of additional surgery.

Videonasopharyngoscopy is performed by introducing a flexible scope through the middle meatus. This instrumental assessment is of para-mount importance for the objective evaluation of the size and location of the VP closure gap. Furthermore, hyponasality (resonance alteration due to nasal airway obstruction) is associated in some cases with VPI and can partially mask an ex-isting hypernasality. The direct visualization of the nasal fossae and the nasopharynx may explain the etiology of hyponasality resulting from obstructive anatomic conditions. This distinction is of partic-ular importance because the type of resonance determines the appropriate treatment. Videonaso-pharyngoscopy has been recognized as superior to videofluoroscopy in identifying small closure gaps and confirming the size of opening, important for surgical planning.[26] It is well tolerated, also by children, provided a flexible endoscope, with diameter inferior to 3 mm, is used. The new tech-nology of microchip videoendoscopes allows high-definition videos to be obtained even with en-doscopes of very small diameter.

In relation to the aforementioned considerations and depending on the nasopharyngeal gap closure, patients are rated according to a 5-point scale[23]: 0 = complete VP closure; 1 = inconstant gap demonstrated by mucus bubbling; 2 = gap involving less than 25% of the VP port at rest; 3 = gap involving 25% to 50% of the VP port; 4 = severe gap involving more than 50% of the VP port. Patients with gaps 1 to 3 (50% of the VP port) are considered candidates for VP fat injection, whereas patients showing a severe gap, rated as 4, are the best candidates for pharyngoplasties (**Table 1**).[7–9]

SURGICAL TECHNIQUE
Anesthesia

The procedure is carried out under general anesthesia.

Fat Harvesting

Fat is usually harvested from the abdomen, although in thin patients fat is obtained from the inner knee or inner thigh. The area is infiltrated with 2.0% mepivacaine with a 1:100,000 epinephrine solution. A stab incision is performed in the lower pole of the umbilicus using a #11 blade. A 2-mm, 3-hole blunt cannula connected to a 10-mL Luer-lock syringe is used. To provide negative pressure, the plunger of the syringe is retracted and maintained in position by means of a towel clamp. Once the necessary amount of fat is harvested, the incision of the umbilicus is sutured with a 5-0 nylon suture, and an elastic garment is placed in the donor area to avoid possible hematoma formation. The lipoaspirate is centrifuged according to the Coleman technique. Fatty layer is transferred to a 3.0-mL Luer-lock syringe using a Luer-lock to Luer-lock adapter.

Fat Placement

The patient is positioned supine with a towel roll placed behind the shoulders to extend the neck. Endotracheal intubation is initiated. A Dingman mouth gag, suspended on a horizontal stand, facilitates exposure and depresses the tongue.

Placement represents the critical step of the procedure, and should be performed with utmost care. A Nelaton probe is inserted into each nostril and passed through the corresponding choana into the mouth. The two heads of the probe are tied together so that the velum is gently retracted superiorly (**Fig. 1**). Thus, the area where adipocytes have to be injected for improving the contact between the velum and the posterior pharyngeal wall is exposed.

Assistance of Endoscope

The assistance of a 70° Storz 4-mm rigid nasal endoscope connected to a video camera and a monitor is used to better visualize the nasopharynx and make the insertion precise (**Fig. 2**).

Fat Injection into the Pharyngeal Walls

Two stab incisions are performed on the posterior pharyngeal wall, at the level of the odontoid process, 5 mm laterally with respect to the midline, on both sides, with an 18-gauge needle or #11 blade. In the past a 19-gauge cannula was used for fat placement, whereby fat often oozed out from the entry point. Nowadays the authors prefer a 21-gauge, 60-mm long disposable malleable microcannula (Thiebaud Medical, Margencel, France), bent as needed. The entry point is small and the risk that fat oozes out is greatly reduced. The cannula is advanced in a cephalad and oblique direction to reach the axis, and continues on a more lateral approach toward the ipsilateral pharyngeal wall in the submucosal plane. However, if an excessive resistance is encountered while injecting fat, with the 3.0-mL syringe a lipoinjection dosage handle (Medicon Instrumente, Tüttlingen, Germany) facilitates the release of fat (see **Fig. 2**).

Level of Placement into the Posterior Pharyngeal Wall

The level of infiltration is of paramount importance. Direct videoendoscopic assistance is critical for assessing the position of the cannula, the injection site, and the amount of fat released. The parcels of

Table 1
Treatment planning according to the degree of VP closure gap as seen at video nasopharyngoscopy

VP Closure Gap	Rating	Treatment
Complete closure	0	None
Mucus bubbling	1	VP fat injection
Gap <25%	2	VP fat injection
Gap 25%–50%	3	Multiple VP fat injections or pharyngoplasty
Gap >50%	4	Pharyngoplasty

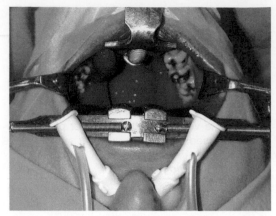

Fig. 1. A Nelaton probe inserted into each nostril and passed into the mouth is gently retracted for good visualization of the nasopharynx, where fat has to be placed. A Dingman mouth gag facilitates exposure and depresses the tongue.

fatty tissue should be injected anterior to the prevertebral fascia within the fibers of the superior constrictor muscle (**Fig. 3**), and not behind the prevertebral fascia, in the loose space that exists immediately anterior to the bodies of the vertebrae (**Fig. 4**). Injecting fat into this space potentially

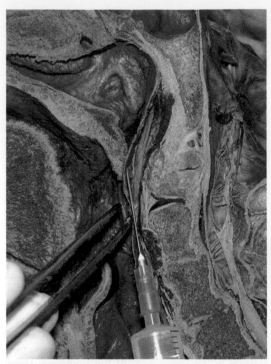

Fig. 3. Cadaveric dissection showing the correct fat injection site, anterior to the prevertebral fascia, within the fibers of the superior constrictor muscle.

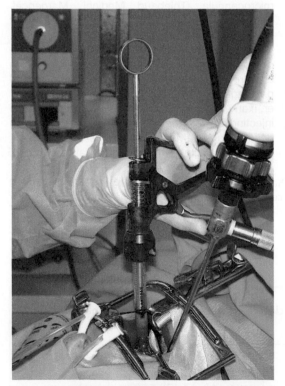

Fig. 2. The assistance of a 70° Storz 4-mm rigid nasal endoscope connected to a video camera and a monitor facilitates nasopharynx exposure for placing fat precisely.

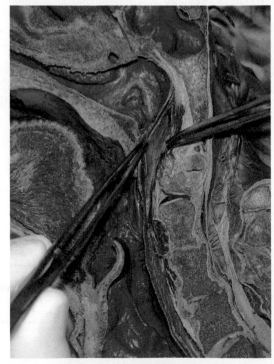

Fig. 4. Cadaveric dissection showing the loose space immediately anterior to the bodies of the vertebrae behind the prevertebral fascia, where fat should decidedly not be injected.

results in dislocation of the graft caudally, along the natural cleavage plane. The cadaveric dissection clearly illustrates this important detail. Numerous tunnels are made to maximize the contact between graft and host tissue. Micro fat parcels are released in multiple directions on withdrawal using the "spaghetti like technique."[33]

Blunt Cannulas

As will become clear, it is mandatory to use blunt cannulas only, never sharp needles, to prevent the possibility of injecting fat into the vessels or injury to the internal carotid artery, which courses laterally, but which could be more medially deviated, as occurs in the velocardiofacial syndrome.[27,28]

Amount of Injected Fat

An average of 2 mL of fat is injected per side. The entry points are sutured with a 5-0 absorbable suture, if needed.

Fat Injection into the Soft Palate

When management of the nasopharyngeal area is completed, fat is injected into the velum and particularly along the midline on the nasal aspect of the uvula (**Fig. 5**) with the goal of softening the scars, frequently present here as a result of previous cleft palate procedure, or creating a bulge that

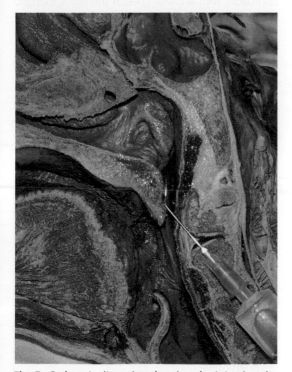

Fig. 5. Cadaveric dissection showing the injection site into the nasal aspect of the uvula.

improves the contact between the velum and the posterior pharyngeal wall. Three stab incisions are made on the velum, the first one being on nasal surface of the uvula and the posterior pillars. If the midline velar scar is particularly stiff, scar release is carried out using an 18-gauge sharp needle with continuous clockwise and counterclockwise movements. Fat is then inserted in the plane between the nasal and oral mucosa. The second stab incision is made at the level of the arch of the tonsillar fossa. An average of 2 mL of fat is injected. The same amount is placed on the contralateral side.

Special Case

In patients affected by submucous cleft, suture of the congenitally separated heads of the levator muscle and fat injection is performed simultaneously to improve the results. The technique is as follows. A 25-mm incision is made along the midline of the palate at the junction between the velum and the hard palate. The area of the posterior nasal spine is exposed. The levator muscle bundles attached to the posterior nasal spine and to the palatal plate are identified, released with a blunt dissector, retropositioned, and sutured end to end at the midline with interrupted 4-0 nylon sutures. Concurrent fat injection is carried out at the 4 walls of the VP port to improve the results obtained by the levator sling suturing and to achieve velopharyngeal competence by creating a bulge in the posterior pharyngeal wall (**Fig. 6**, **Table 2**).

The Problem of Fat Graft Retention

It is well known that transplanted fat undergoes a certain degree of resorption rate, which varies from 20% to 80% depending on numerous factors.[29] For this reason, it is essential that the repeatability of the procedure is indicated in the informed consent, emphasizing that more than 1 surgical session is necessary.

POSTOPERATIVE CARE

No special care is needed. Prophylactic antibiotic treatment is administered in every case.

POTENTIAL COMPLICATIONS

No complications have occurred in the authors' series of patients, none of whom experienced respiratory obstruction after surgery. However, it has been reported that OSA, related to a significant weight gain, may represent a potential risk.[30]

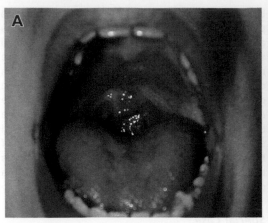
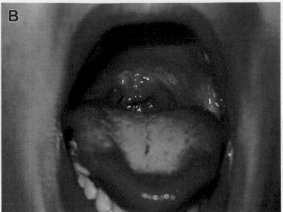

Fig. 6. Submucous cleft with bifid uvula and zona pellucida (case 1). Preoperative view (A) and postoperative view at 1 year after levator sling reconstruction concurrent with fat injection (B).

CASE EXAMPLES

Case 1: **Fig. 6**, **Table 2**
Case 2: **Fig. 7**, **Table 3**
Case 3: **Fig. 8**, **Table 4**, Video 1

DISCUSSION

Surgical management of VPI aims at improving voice resonance and correcting nasal air escape by restoring a competent velopharyngeal sphincter. It is therefore critical to select patients properly, so as to choose the most effective procedure. Assessment of VPI requires the examination of multiple variables from perceptual evaluation of speech intelligibility to aerodynamic assessment of nasal air escape. The key point for surgical planning is the dynamic study of the VP port movements during speech and the quantification of the closure gap, using flexible videonasoendoscopy and/or videofluoroscopy.

Mild to moderate VPI, the so-called borderline conditions with minimal nasal air escape, constitute a true dilemma for surgeons. Pharyngoplasty represents an overtreatment, potentially causing permanent sequelae such as respiratory obstruction, snoring, and OSA. Augmentation of the posterior pharyngeal wall using the currently available biomaterials is often unsuccessful. Reabsorbable implants vanish within a few months, whereas permanent implants may migrate, extrude, or give rise to foreign body reactions.[13–17] Commonly, the wait-and-see approach, with endless speech therapies focused on improved oral articulation and increased velar strengthening, is the typical decision. On calculating the risk-to-benefit ratio of the aforementioned major procedures, often these patients are not considered good candidates for additional surgery.

Autologous fat grafting to reduce the passage between the oropharynx and nasopharynx offers several advantages to the patient: morbidity is considerably less, anatomy of the pharyngeal walls

Table 2
Case example

	Patient Characteristics	Age at Evaluation (y)	Type of Procedure	No. of Fat Injection Sessions (Amount Injected)	Result
Case 1 (see **Fig. 6**)	Submucous cleft (type 2, see **Table 1**)	11	Levator sling reconstruction and fat injection into the velum and pharyngeal walls	1 (5.0 mL)	Improved nasal air escape

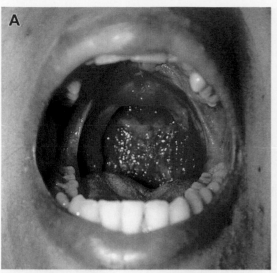 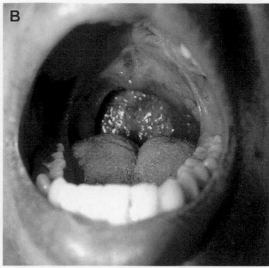

Fig. 7. Sequela of cleft palate repair with retracted scars (case 2). Preoperative view (*A*) and postoperative view at 5 months (*B*), with softened scars.

is not altered, the procedure can be repeated if necessary, and the postoperative course is irrelevant.

Fat injection is usually considered a safe operation, provided that some basic principles are respected.

Knowledge of Head and Neck Anatomy

As a general rule, surgery requires clear knowledge of anatomy. In dealing with the head and neck structures this rule is even more evident.

Never Sharp Needles; Blunt Cannulas Only

In performing this procedure it is mandatory to use blunt cannulas only and thus avoid the risk of injecting fat into the pharyngeal vessels or into the carotid artery, which courses laterally in the pharynx. In 2010 a dramatic event occurred in a British Hospital, when small amounts of fat (0.2–0.3 mL), injected in the posterior and lateral pharyngeal walls for treating VPI in an 18-year-old girl with sequela of the cleft palate, were accidentally introduced into the carotid artery. Instead of a blunt cannula, the surgeon used a 14-gauge needle connected to a 10-mL syringe. Immediately thereafter the patient suffered a massive stroke as a consequence of fat embolism. At 3 years the patient is still aphasic and hemiplegic on the right side, and her left eye is amaurotic (R.F. Mazzola, personal communication, 2013).[31]

Current studies suggest that autologous fat possesses the regenerative potential mediated by the pluripotent stem cells present in its stromal vascular fraction, and this may account for an important role in neoangiogenesis and regeneration of the host tissue.[32]

	Patient Characteristics	Age at Evaluation (y)	Type of Procedure	No. of Fat Injection Sessions (Amount Injected)	Result
Case 2 (see **Fig. 7**)	Sequela of cleft palate repair with retracted scars and nasal air escape (type 2, see **Table 1**)	18	Fat injection into the velum and pharyngeal walls	1 (5.0 mL)	Improved nasal air escape with softened scars

Table 3
Case example

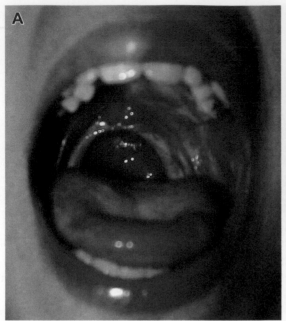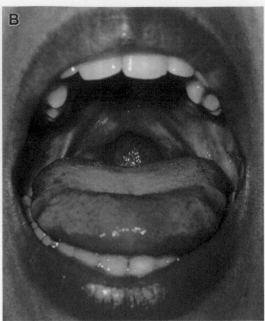

Fig. 8. Sequela of cleft palate repair with retracted scars (case 3). Preoperative view (*A*) and postoperative view at 7 years after 3 sessions of fat injection (*B*), with softened scars.

The Goals of Fat Injection for Velopharyngeal Incompetence

Fat injection for the treatment of VPI fulfills a dual goal. It reduces the existing gap between the oral and nasal cavity, thus ameliorating nasal air escape, and softens scar contractures in cases of VPI secondary to cleft palate repair (see **Figs. 7** and **8**, Video 1). Once the midline scar has been released and has become more pliable, the velum improves its elevation, facilitating its approximation to the posterior pharyngeal wall.

A further advantage of fat injection is the possibility of maintaining the achieved results by repeating fat injections when facial growth takes place, if decompensation of velopharyngeal closure occurs.

Overinjection, or fat bolus, performed in an attempt to further reduce the VP gap, is not considered the appropriate treatment. On the contrary, it is responsible for the formation of oily cysts.[33] The spaghetti-like technique represents the method of choice to maximize surface contact with the host tissue and enhance the survival of fat parcels.[34]

Fat Grafting for Submucous Clefts

Submucous cleft palate is often associated with congenital short palate.[35] Numerous repair strategies, most of them fairly invasive, have been proposed over the years to reduce the risk of postoperative VPI. In the authors' opinion, fat injection concurrent with the suturing of the

Table 4
Case example

	Patient Characteristics	Age at Evaluation (y)	Type of Procedure	No. of Fat Injection Sessions (Amount Injected)	Result
Case 3 (see **Fig. 8**, Video 1)	Sequela of cleft palate repair with retracted scars and nasal air escape (type 2, see **Table 1**)	10	Fat injection into the velum and pharyngeal walls	3 (4.5 + 5.0 + 5.0 mL)	Improved nasal air escape with softened scars

congenitally separated heads of the levator muscle has proved to be useful in gaining palatal length and diminishing the gap between the velum and the posterior pharyngeal wall. This technique represents an innovative procedure that requires further objective analysis.

SUMMARY

Surgical management of VPI aims at improving voice resonance and correcting nasal air escape by restoring a competent VP port. It is therefore critical to select patients properly to determine the most appropriate treatment. Assessment of VPI requires the examination of multiple variables, from perceptual evaluation of speech intelligibility to aerodynamic measurement of nasal air escape. The key point for surgical planning is the dynamic assessment of the VP port movements during speech and the quantification of the closure gap, using flexible videonasoendoscopy and/or videofluoroscopy.

Autologous fat injection represents a minimally invasive alternative to major surgery in the management of mild to moderate VPI, and minimizes the risk of complications and sequelae. It represents a versatile procedure that can be performed in a tailored way, depending on the requirements of each specific case, without modifying the anatomy of the VP port.

SUPPLEMENTARY DATA

Supplementary data related to this article can be found online at http://dx.doi.org/10.1016/j.cps.2015.03.002.

REFERENCES

1. Gart MS, Gosain AK. Surgical management of velopharyngeal insufficiency. Clin Plast Surg 2014;41: 253–70.
2. Sommerlad BC, Mehendale FV, Birch MJ, et al. Palate re-repair revisited. Cleft Palate Craniofac J 2002; 39:295–307.
3. Furlow LT Jr. Cleft palate repair by double opposing Z-plasty. Plast Reconstr Surg 1986;78:724–38.
4. Dorrance GM, Bransfield JW. Push-back operation for repair of cleft palate. Plast Reconstr Surg 1946; 1:145–69.
5. Schönborn K. Über eine neue Methode der Staphylorraphie. Arch Klin Chir 1876;19:527–31.
6. Rosenthal W. Zur Frage der Gaumenplastik. Zbl f Chir 1924;51:1621–7.
7. Sanvenero Rosselli G. La divisione congenita del Labbro e del Palato. Roma (Italy): Pozzi; 1934. p. 262–4.
8. Hynes W. Pharyngoplasty by muscle transplantation. Br J Plast Surg 1950;3:128–35.
9. Orticochea M. Construction of a dynamic muscle sphincter in cleft palates. Plast Reconstr Surg 1968;41:323–7.
10. Gersuny R. Über eine subkutane Prothese. Ztschr f Heilk 1900;21:199–201.
11. Gaza von W. Über freie Fettgewebstransplantation in den retropharyngealen Raum bei Gaumenspalte. Arch Klin Chir 1926;142:590–9.
12. Hagerty RF, Hill MJ. Cartilage pharyngoplasty in cleft palate patients. Surg Gynecol Obstet 1961;112:350–6.
13. Blocksma R. Silicone implants for velopharyngeal incompetence: a progress report. Cleft Palate J 1964;16:72–81.
14. Brauer RO. Retropharyngeal implantation of silicone gel pillows for velopharyngeal incompetence. Plast Reconstr Surg 1973;51:254–62.
15. Lewy RB, Cole L, Wepman J. Teflon injection in the correction of velopharyngeal insufficiency. Ann Otol Rhinol Laryngol 1965;74:847–80.
16. Sturim HS, Jacob CT Jr. Teflon pharyngoplasty. Plast Reconstr Surg 1972;49:180–5.
17. Brigger MT, Ashland JE, Hartnick CJ. Injection pharyngoplasty with calcium hydroxylapatite for velopharyngeal insufficiency: patient selection and technique. Arch Otolaryngol Head Neck Surg 2010;136:666–70.
18. Wardill WE. Cleft palate. Br J Surg 1928;16:127–48.
19. Hess DA, Hagerty RF, Mylin WK. Velar motility, velopharyngeal closure, and speech proficiency in cartilage pharyngoplasty: an eight year study. Cleft Palate J 1968;5:153–62.
20. Bardot J, Salazard B, Casanova D, et al. Les séquélles vélopharyngées dans le fentes labioalvéolopalatovélaires: pharyngoplastie par lipostructure du pharynx. Rev Stomatol Chir Maxillofac 2007;108:352–6.
21. Leuchter I, Schweizer V, Hohlfeld J, et al. Treatment of velopharyngeal insufficiency by autologous fat injection. Eur Arch Otorhinolaryngol 2010;267:977–83.
22. Cantarella G, Mazzola RF, Mantovani M, et al. Treatment of velopharyngeal insufficiency by pharyngeal and velar fat injections. Otolaryngol Head Neck Surg 2011;145:401–3.
23. Cantarella G, Mazzola RF, Mantovani M, et al. Fat injections for the treatment of velopharyngeal insufficiency. J Craniofac Surg 2012;23:634–7.
24. Filip C, Matzen M, Aagenæs I, et al. Autologous fat transplantation to the velopharynx for treating persistent velopharyngeal insufficiency of mild degree secondary to overt or submucous cloft palate. J Plast Reconstr Aesthet Surg 2013;66: 337–44.
25. Bishop A, Hong P, Bezuhly M. Autologous fat grafting for the treatment of velopharyngeal insufficiency: state of the art. J Plast Reconstr Aesthet Surg 2014; 67:1–8.

26. Lam DJ, Starr JR, Perkins JA, et al. A comparison of nasoendoscopy and multiview videofluoroscopy in assessing velopharyngeal insufficiency. Otolaryngol Head Neck Surg 2006;134:394–402.

27. Oppenheimer AG, Fulmer S, Shifteh K, et al. Cervical vascular and upper airway asymmetry in velo-cardio-facial syndrome: correlation of nasopharyngoscopy with MRA. Int J Pediatr Otorhinolaryngol 2010;74:619–25.

28. Baek RM, Koo YT, Kim SJ, et al. Internal carotid artery variations in velocardiofacial syndrome patients and its implications for surgery. Plast Reconstr Surg 2013;132:806e–10e.

29. Kølle SF, Fischer-Nielsen A, Mathiasen AB, et al. Enrichment of autologous fat grafts with ex-vivo expanded adipose tissue-derived stem cells for graft survival: a randomised placebo-controlled trial. Lancet 2013;382:1113–20.

30. Teixeira RP, Reid JA, Greensmith A. Fatty hypertrophy cause obstructive sleep apnea after fat injection for velopharyngeal incompetence. Cleft Palate Craniofac J 2011;48:473–7.

31. Filip C. Response re: "Autologous fat grafting for the treatment of velopharyngeal insufficiency: state of the art". J Plast Reconstr Aesthet Surg 2014;67: 1155–6.

32. Fraser JK, Zhu M, Wulur I, et al. Adipose-derived stem cells. Methods Mol Biol 2008;449:59–67.

33. Eto H, Kato H, Suga H, et al. The fate of adipocytes after nonvascularized fat grafting: evidence of early death and replacement of adipocytes. Plast Reconstr Surg 2012;129:1081–92.

34. Kato H, Mineda K, Eto H, et al. Degeneration, regeneration, and cicatrization after fat grafting: dynamic total tissue remodeling during the first 3 months. Plast Reconstr Surg 2014;133: 303e–13e.

35. Weatherley-White RC, Sakura CY Jr, Brenner LD, et al. Submucous cleft palate. Its incidence, natural history, and indications for treatment. Plast Reconstr Surg 1972;49:297–304.

Percutaneous Aponeurotomy and Lipofilling (PALF)
A Regenerative Approach to Dupuytren Contracture

Steven E.R. Hovius, MD, PhD[a],*, Hester J. Kan, MD[a],
Jennifer S.N. Verhoekx, MD, PhD[a], Roger K. Khouri, MD[b]

KEYWORDS

- Dupuytren disease • Fat grafting • Lipofilling • Minimally invasive • Needle fasciotomy
- Needle aponeurotomy

KEY POINTS

- Extensive percutaneous aponeurotomy and lipofilling (PALF) is a minimally invasive surgical technique. No incisions are made, no tissue is removed, and no sutures are used.
- Patients are able to return to normal activities after a median of 9 days. The technique is safe. Due instead of owing to the strong extension force applied on the contracture, the needle tip selectively severs the cords placed under tension while the looser neurovascular bundles are spared. Lipofilling restores the subdermal fat deficiency, which is an inherent part of the pathology of Dupuytren contracture.
- Adipose-derived-stem cells (ADSCs) in the lipoaspirate may inhibit proliferation of the contractile myofibroblast.
- When comparing PALF with limited fasciectomy (LF), no significant differences are observed in overall postoperative contracture correction and in recurrence of the contractures within 1 year follow-up.

INTRODUCTION

Dupuytren disease (DD) is a chronic progressive fibroproliferative disease characterized by flexion contractures of the digits, especially the metacarpophalangeal (MP)-joint and proximal interphalangeal (PIP) joints.[1] In DD, the formation of palmar nodules have classically been described as the first sign of the disease, which are the result of myofibroblast proliferation and extracellular matrix synthesis.[2] Myofibroblasts are the cells responsible for the development of the disease. In the later stages of DD, nodules mature to form collagen-rich, acellular fibrotic cords, which lead to digital contractures.

The disease is more prevalent in the Northern part of Europe. Males are more affected than females, and it is more common in older patients.[3,4] Family predisposition and genetic pathways are described for DD.[5] Other factors such as smoking, alcohol consumption, manual work, hand trauma, diabetes, and epilepsy have also been linked to DD.[6–8] Factors that contribute to the severity of the disease, also known as diathesis, are (1) bilateral hand involvement, (2) ectopic disease, (3) family members with DD, and (4) early onset of the disease. In patients with severe diathesis, the disease is more likely to recur after treatment.[9]

[a] Department of Plastic and Reconstructive Surgery, Erasmus University Medical Center, Dr Molewaterplein 50-60, 3015 GE Rotterdam, The Netherlands; [b] Miami Hand Center, 2750 SW 37th Avenue, Miami, FL, USA
* Corresponding author.
E-mail address: s.e.r.hovius@erasmusmc.nl

Clin Plastic Surg 42 (2015) 375–381
http://dx.doi.org/10.1016/j.cps.2015.03.006

Many treatment options are available to treat the symptoms of DD. Established flexion contractures are most commonly treated by surgical excision of the cord through a limited fasciectomy (LF). Complications after surgical treatment include pain, edema, paresthesia, infections, hematoma, nerve lesions, arterial lesions, tendon ruptures, and chronic regional pain syndromes (CRPSs). The overall cumulative complication rate for LF reported in a randomized controlled trial was 30%.[10] Recently, a 20.9% recurrence rate 5 years postsurgery has been described for LF.[11]

The prolonged postoperative recovery of the LF has led to a trend toward minimally invasive techniques in the past 10 years. These techniques include needle aponeurotomy (NA) and collagenase injections, which enzymatically digest and weaken the cord.[12–14] These minimally invasive methods are gaining more popularity as treatment of DD, despite the higher recurrence rates associated with them.[11,15]

In an attempt to overcome the high recurrence rates after NA, the authors' group is investigating a new treatment strategy, a more extensive percutaneous aponeurotomy that is performed while maintaining the cord under tension followed by lipofilling of the loosened structure. The grafted lipoaspirate is known to contain stem cells, and there is now increasing evidence that stem cells may be used to treat fibrotic diseases.[16–19] The authors' study showed that ADSCs inhibit proliferation of the contractile myofibroblasts and mediate these effects by soluble factors, influenced by cell contact.[20] Myofibroblasts are the key cells leading to the development of fibrosis and flexion contractures in DD.[21] Therefore, inhibiting myofibroblasts using a lipoaspirate containing ADSCs represents a rational treatment strategy for DD.

Furthermore, DD is associated with subdermal fat deficiency and atrophy as the pathologic fibrosis displaces the fat.[22] Fat grafting is able to restore the loss of this important padding. Fat has already been used in the early twentieth century to infiltrate the diseased area in an attempt to treat flexion contractures of the digits.[23] As fat grafting has gained popularity over the past decade, the authors reintroduced this procedure for DD. Their findings lend support to the potential benefit of lipofilling in conjunction with an extensive needle fasciotomy of the cord as a new strategy in the treatment of DD.

TREATMENT GOALS AND PLANNED OUTCOMES

DD is a chronic progressive disease, and all currently available treatments only address the symptoms rather than treating the underlying pathologic condition. Therefore the goals are to maximally straighten the finger, to shorten the convalescence period and to delay recurrence with a minimum of complications. Outcome measures are therefore patient satisfaction, convalescence period, and objective measurements of range of motion and of contracture recurrence.

PREOPERATIVE PLANNING AND PREPARATION

The procedure is ideally suited for patients who want to minimize recovery time. A great advantage of this new technique is its ability to treat multidigital ray disease in one session, where conventional open surgery would require extensive dissection of every ray through multiple stages.

Younger patients, especially women, with severe diathesis or with recurrent PIP joint contractures are less-ideal candidates. Long-standing PIP joint contractures are difficult to release fully with this technique because of inherent joint contracture and attenuation of the extensor tendon central slip. The authors advise not to treat patients who had previous surgery with flaps in the affected area because the scarred neurovascular bundles are no longer loose and therefore are as vulnerable to be severed by the needle as the recurrent cord and the surrounding scar tissue.

To treat the cords and nodules and to free the affected skin from the underlying pathologic process, a 19-gauge needle and a malleable semirigid hand retractor is needed. After infiltration of the designated liposuction donor area (typically the abdomen) with a mixture of 500 mL of 0.9% NaCl, 20 mL lidocaine, and 0.5 mg epinephrine and bicarbonate, a syringe liposuction using a blunt tip cannula with multiple holes is performed. Patients can be treated either in an outpatient clinic with proper facilities or in day care. Anesthesia can be provided in the following ways: (1) locoregional block for the upper extremity combined with local anesthesia for the liposuction area, (2) general anesthesia, (3) peripheral isolated or combined nerve block together with local anesthesia for the liposuction area, and (4) local superficial anesthesia of the affected fingers combined with local anesthesia for the liposuction area.

The duration of the minimal invasive procedure depends on the number of digital rays involved and the extent of the disease and typically requires the same operative time as LF.

PATIENT POSITIONING

Patients are placed in the supine position with the affected arm placed on an arm table.

PROCEDURAL APPROACH

After complete exsanguination, the affected hand with the digital contractures is placed under maximal tension of the rather stiff malleable hand retractor (**Fig. 1**). Starting from proximal to distal, in an orderly manner, a series of multiple palmar punctures are made with a 19-gauge needle along the entire length of the palpable cord (see **Fig. 1**A). The needle pricks are staggered 2 to 3 mm apart, and the release of an entire digital ray often requires 20 to 30 pricks or more. To prevent damage to the digital arteries and nerves, it is important to gauge the depth of needle penetration, which should be kept less than 2 to 3 mm proximal to the transverse palmar crease, while beyond that level, the maximal depth becomes 1 to 1.5 mm, depending on the thickness of the patient's skin. The bevel of the needle can be used to gauge the appropriate depth. By continuously providing maximal tension as the contracture is released, the small nicks are more likely to cut the tight cords than the looser neurovascular bundles. The looser neurovascular bundles tend to divert, whereas the taut cords snap like a tight violin string. Furthermore, because

of the inherently spiral woven structure of the fibrous cord, multiple superficial nicks along its length are sufficient to destroy it by attrition.

It is imperative to keep the contracted digits under tension when working along a wide area around the contracture. Tension is crucial to the selective cutting of the needle, and it allows the surgeon to localize the residual restricting bands by palpation. Skin pits caused by deep full-thickness skin retractions into the subcutaneous tissue are released by severing the diseased fibers that insert into the dermis using a horizontal windshield wiper motion of the needle in a plane just below the skin (see **Fig. 1**B).

The extension of the digits and the tension is constantly adjusted till the contracture is fully released and the nodules become soft. With a blunt-tip 14-gauge cannula, the gravity-sedimented lipoaspirate harvested from the flanks or abdomen is diffusely injected through 2 to 3 needle entry sites in the palm and the digit. Normally, a total of 10 mL of very loose only decanted lipoaspirate per digital ray is injected. Some of the lipofilling escapes through the needle release sites. Furthermore, because the injected fat is

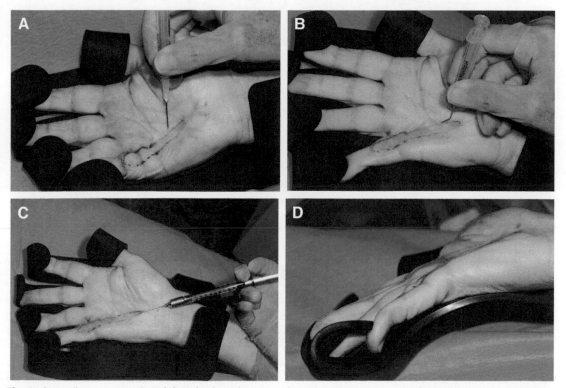

Fig. 1. Operation room setting: (*A*) multiple nicks are made with a 19-gauge needle from proximal to distal; (*B*) a hooked needle is used to release the skin from the underlying tissue; (*C*) fat is injected when the cord is fully released; (*D*) end position after fat grafting.

very dilute, some ballooning of the palmar skin is afforded (see **Fig. 1**C). By placing the skin folds and pits under tension, this tumescence also facilitates their release with the needle (see **Fig. 1**D). Two case examples are provided with MP joint and PIP joint contractures with long-term follow-up (**Figs. 2** and **3**).

POTENTIAL COMPLICATIONS AND THEIR MANAGEMENT

Over the past 7 years, between Miami and Rotterdam, the authors have treated over 300 patients with DD using the PALF procedure described above. They have had only one permanent nerve

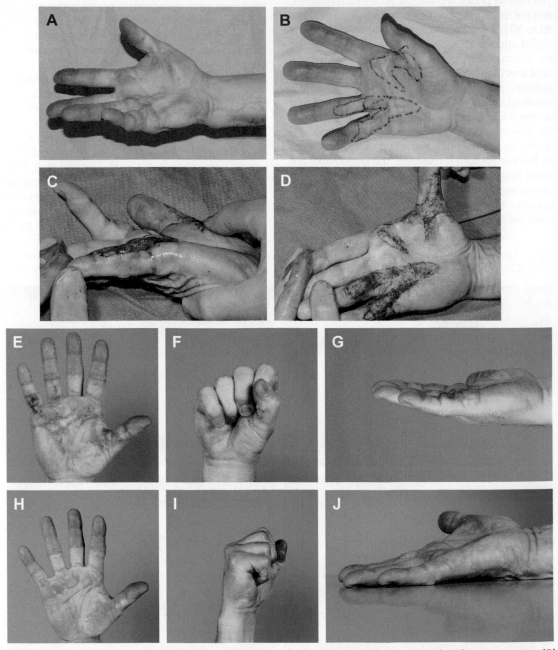

Fig. 2. Patient example: (*A*) affected hand; (*B*) drawing of affected area; (*C*) rays treated with extensive NA; (*D*) hand treated with PALF; (*E*) 2 weeks post-PALF stretched fingers palmar view; (*F*) 2 weeks post-PALF ability of making a full fist; (*G*) 2 weeks post-PALF stretched fingers lateral view; (*H*) 1 year post-PALF; (*I*) 1 year post-PALF ability of making a full fist; (*J*) 1 year post-PALF full finger extension.

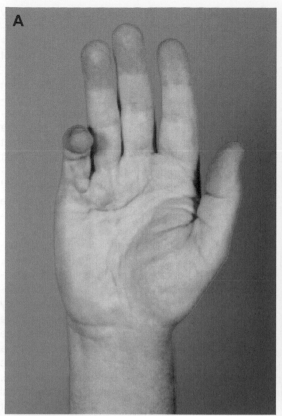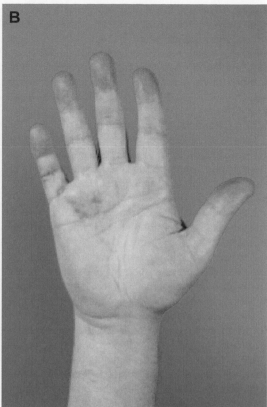

Fig. 3. Patient example: (*A*) severe PIP contracture of the small finger; (*B*) 2-year follow-up of same patient, note absent scarring and fat padding at the fifth ray.

lesion, two transient neuropraxias, and four CRPS cases; one tendon rupture was seen, which required an additional operation. Also, one patient had an infection, which resolved with antibiotics. Overall, the complication rate was very low considering that the authors were often dealing with severe contractures that would have almost always required multiple Z-plasty flaps or skin grafts.

POSTPROCEDURAL CARE

During surgery a plaster extension splint is incorporated in the dressing on the operated hand. After 5 to 7 days, the splint is removed at the outpatient clinic and the patient is allowed to return to normal activities. The patients have no sutures to be removed and no incision to heal, only signs of already healed needle pricks.

REHABILITATION AND RECOVERY

The authors advise patients to use a night extension splint for 4 months and to visit a hand therapist should there be any stiffness.

DISCUSSION

During follow-up at the outpatient clinic, we found that the patients had supple subcutaneous fat pads. Lipofilling restores the subdermal fat deficiency and restores normal pliability, which is rarely seen in the scarred hand after LF because the palmar skin stays tethered.

In the study published in 2011, the authors described 50 patients with complete preoperative and postoperative data and a mean follow-up of 44 weeks. In this retrospective study, a significant flexion contracture correction from 61° to 27° for the PIP joint and from 37° to –5° for the MP joint was accomplished; 88% of the patients achieved a Tubiana stage 1 after surgery. A total of 91 patients were treated, and 87 (95%) were highly satisfied and would recommend the operation to family and friends. Most patients returned to either work or vocational activities within 2 to 4 weeks.[24]

In 2010, the authors started a randomized controlled trial at the Erasmus University Medical Center (Rotterdam, The Netherlands) to compare LF with PALF. Preliminary results reveal the same contracture correction after surgery for the PALF group and the LF group. At 1-year follow-up, there was no difference in the recurrence of the contractures between the standard LF and the PALF techniques. Recurrence rates are difficult to provide, because these results depend considerably on the definitions used to describe recurrence. The authors have reviewed the different definitions used for recurrence of DD and conducted a Delphi study among experts to acquire a broad supported definition of recurrence in DD.[25]

The most striking difference, however, was in the satisfaction and the convalescence rate; on the average, patients who had undergone PALF were able to return to normal use of the hand within 9 days compared with 17 days for the LF-treated patients. Furthermore, the authors were able to release the tightest contractures without recourse to flaps or grafts.

Concerning indication, the first author does not use PALF if many operations have been performed on the same ray, especially if the patient already experiences sensory and/or circulatory disturbances of the involved finger from a previous operation. Furthermore, in a young patient with a severe diathesis, this technique is not advocated. However, PALF is preferred in older patients and also in patients with multiple rays involved, even with severe contractures. PALF can also be used if patients have been operated once before, but without sensory disturbances in the involved fingers.

with faster recovery, less complications, and very high patient satisfaction. Even in case of recurrence, the procedure can be repeated with minimal morbidity and rapid return to normal use of the hand.

After extensive percutaneous NA with disruption of the affected tissue, aggregates of myofibroblasts remain and are likely to rebuild the contracture. Subsequent lipofilling in the affected area results in a reduction of density and cell contact of contractile myofibroblasts. ADSC's in the graft inhibit the proliferation of the contractile myofibroblast to limit the progression of DD. The authors' preliminary results suggest that this extensive PALF procedure has a positive effect on the recurrence rate.

PALF is a radical departure from the conventional excisional surgery. Instead of removing, the fibrosis is treated by adding tissue with regenerative potential. Instead of the complication-prone flaps, the contracture is released by percutaneous mesh expansion of the restrictive fascia.[26] The procedure selectively disrupts the pathologic cords and turns their fibers into a recipient scaffold for regenerative fat grafts capable of altering the pathologic condition. PALF is a regenerative alternative to traditional excisional surgery and flaps in the treatment of DD.

CLINICAL RESULTS IN THE LITERATURE

Retrospective study • PIP joint: 61°–27° • MP joint: 37° to –5° • 95.6% of the patients were highly satisfied	Hovius et al,[24]	Journal of Plastic and Reconstructive Surgery (PRS)	2011
Prospective controlled randomized study • Same overall contracture correction after surgery for the PALF group and the LF group • No difference in recurrent contractures within 1 year • Return to normal use of hand within 8 days for PALF vs 17 days for LF	Kan et al,[25]	Journal of Plastic Reconstructive and Aesthetic Surgery	2015

SUMMARY

The PALF procedure is introduced as a new treatment alternative for DD that is safe, minimally invasive, and at least as effective as the standard LF

REFERENCES

1. McFarlane R, McGrouther DA, Flint MH, editors. Dupuytren's disease. Edinburgh (United Kingdom): Churchill Livingstone; 1990.

2. Luck JV. Dupuytren's contracture; a new concept of the pathogenesis correlated with surgical management. J Bone Joint Surg Am 1959;41-A(4): 635–64.

3. Lanting R, van den Heuvel ER, Westerink B, et al. Prevalence of Dupuytren disease in The Netherlands. Plast Reconstr Surg 2013;132(2):394–403 [Comparative Study Research Support, Non-U.S. Gov't].

4. Mikkelsen OA. The prevalence of Dupuytren's disease in Norway. A study in a representative population sample of the municipality of Haugesund. Acta Chir Scand 1972;138(7):695–700.

5. Dolmans GH, Werker PM, Hennies HC, et al. Wnt signaling and Dupuytren's disease. N Engl J Med 2011;365(4):307–17 [Research Support, Non-U.S. Gov't].

6. Lanting R, Broekstra DC, Werker PM, et al. A systematic review and meta-analysis on the prevalence of Dupuytren disease in the general population of Western countries. Plast Reconstr Surg 2014; 133(3):593–603 [Meta-Analysis Research Support, Non-U.S. Gov't Review].

7. Geoghegan JM, Forbes J, Clark DI, et al. Dupuytren's disease risk factors. J Hand Surg Br 2004 Oct;29(5):423–6.

8. Degreef I, De Smet L. Risk factors in Dupuytren's diathesis: is recurrence after surgery predictable? Acta Orthop Belg 2011;77(1):27–32.

9. Abe Y, Rokkaku T, Ofuchi S, et al. An objective method to evaluate the risk of recurrence and extension of Dupuytren's disease. J Hand Surg 2004; 29(5):427–30 [Comparative Study].

10. van Rijssen AL, Gerbrandy FS, Ter Linden H, et al. A comparison of the direct outcomes of percutaneous needle fasciotomy and limited fasciectomy for Dupuytren's disease: a 6-week follow-up study. J Hand Surg Am 2006;31(5):717–25.

11. van Rijssen AL, Ter Linden H, Werker PM. 5-year results of randomized clinical trial on treatment in Dupuytren's disease: percutaneous needle fasciotomy versus limited fasciectomy. Plast Reconstr Surg 2012;129:469–77.

12. Hurst LC, Badalamente MA, Hentz VR, et al. Injectable collagenase Clostridium histolyticum for Dupuytren's contracture. N Engl J Med 2009;361(10): 968–79.

13. Starkweather KD, Lattuga S, Hurst LC, et al. Collagenase in the treatment of Dupuytren's disease: an in vitro study. J Hand Surg 1996;21(3):490–5 [In Vitro Research Support, Non-U.S. Gov't].

14. Foucher G, Medina J, Malizos K. Percutaneous needle fasciotomy in Dupuytren disease. Tech Hand Up Extrem Surg 2001;5(3):161–4.

15. Watt AJ, Curtin CM, Hentz VR. Collagenase injection as nonsurgical treatment of Dupuytren's disease: 8-year follow-up. J Hand Surg 2010;35(4):534–9, 539.e1. [Clinical Trial, Phase II Randomized Controlled Trial].

16. Castiglione F, Hedlund P, Van der Aa F, et al. Intratunical injection of human adipose tissue-derived stem cells prevents fibrosis and is associated with improved erectile function in a rat model of Peyronie's disease. Eur Urol 2013;63(3):551–60 [Research Support, Non-U.S. Gov't].

17. Alfarano C, Roubeix C, Chaaya R, et al. Intraparenchymal injection of bone marrow mesenchymal stem cells reduces kidney fibrosis after ischemia-reperfusion in cyclosporine-immunosuppressed rats. Cell Transplant 2012;21(9):2009–19 [Research Support, Non-U.S. Gov't].

18. Zhao W, Li JJ, Cao DY, et al. Intravenous injection of mesenchymal stem cells is effective in treating liver fibrosis. World J Gastroenterol 2012;18(10):1048–58 [Research Support, Non-U.S. Gov't].

19. Elnakish MT, Kuppusamy P, Khan M. Stem cell transplantation as a therapy for cardiac fibrosis. J Pathol 2013;229(2):347–54 [Research Support, Non-U.S. Gov't Review].

20. Verhoekx JS, Mudera V, Walbeehm ET, et al. Adipose-derived stem cells inhibit the contractile myofibroblast in Dupuytren's disease. Plast Reconstr Surg 2013;132(5):1139–48.

21. Tomasek JJ, Gabbiani G, Hinz B, et al. Myofibroblasts and mechano-regulation of connective tissue remodelling. Nat Rev Mol Cell Biol 2002;3(5):349–63 [Research Support, Non-U.S. Gov't Research Support, U.S. Gov't, P.H.S. Review].

22. Rayan GM. Clinical presentation and types of Dupuytren's disease. Hand Clin 1999;15(1):87–96. vii. [Case Reports Review].

23. Lexer E. Die Freie fettransplantation. In: Die Transplantation Teil 1, Stuttgart, Ferdinand Ecke. 1919. p. 265–302.

24. Hovius SE, Kan HJ, Smit X, et al. Extensive percutaneous aponeurotomy and lipografting: a new treatment for Dupuytren disease. Plast Reconstr Surg 2011;128(1):221–8.

25. Kan HJ, Verrijp FW, Huisstede BM, et al. The consequences of different definitions for recurrence of Dupuytren's disease [review]. J Plast Reconstr Aesthet Surg 2015;66(1):95–103.

26. Khouri RK, Smit JM, Cardoso E, et al. Percutaneous aponeurotomy and lipofilling: a regenerative alternative to flap reconstruction? Plast Reconstr Surg 2013;132(5):1280–90 [Case Reports].

Complications of Fat Grafting
How They Occur and How to Find, Avoid, and Treat Them

Kotaro Yoshimura, MD[a],*, Sydney R. Coleman, MD[b]

KEYWORDS

- Fat grafting • Adipose-derived stem/stromal cell • Tissue necrosis • Oil cyst • Calcification
- Blindness • Infection

KEY POINTS

- Blindness and stroke have occurred as a result of arterial injection of fat tissue in almost every part of the face. The injection of large boluses and the use of sharp needles/cannulas should be avoided in the face.
- Most of the common complications such as no/minimal graft retention, infection, oil cysts, and calcifications are related to necrosis of grafted fat. To minimize fat necrosis, surgeons should optimize each step from liposuction to lipoinjection. Injection as small aliquots/noodles of fat (preferably 2 mm in diameter) is particularly important.
- Although fat grafting is a minimally invasive surgical procedure, surgeons have to be cautious to avoid any unexpected damage to the donor and recipient sites to minimize the perioperative risk and complications.

INTRODUCTION

Recent technical and scientific advances in fat grafting procedures and concepts have improved predictability of fat grafting. Large-volume fat injection is gaining much attention as an attracting procedure for body contouring and reconstruction, but an increasing number of complications also has been recognized over the world.[1] In this article, typical complications after fat grafting are described, as well as an explanation of how and why they occur, and how surgeons can avoid and treat complications.

COMPLICATIONS AFTER FAT GRAFTING PROCEDURES

Most of the common complications are related to necrosis of grafted fat, which can be minimized by technical improvements, but there are rare but catastrophic complications such as blindness and stroke.[2] Typical complications and possible complaints by patients will be discussed.

Embolization: Blindness, Strokes, and Skin/Tissue Necrosis

Probably the most devastating potential complication of fat grafting is embolization after intravascular injection. Blindness from a fat injection was first reported in 1988.[3] Few details were given, but the basic presentation was identical to the later reports. The patient experienced excruciating pain accompanied by immediate and permanent loss of vision in 1 eye. There have been reports of permanent unilateral blindness from central retinal artery occlusion by fat grafting, frequently

Financial Disclosure: Authors report no commercial associations or financial disclosures with regard to this article.
[a] Department of Plastic Surgery, School of Medicine, University of Tokyo, 7-3-1 Hongo, Bunkyo-Ku, Tokyo 113-8655, Japan; [b] Department of Plastic Surgery, New York University Langone Medical Center, New York, NY, USA
* Corresponding author.
E-mail address: kotaro-yoshimura@umin.ac.jp

accompanying stroke and skin necrosis. Although most instances of central retinal artery occlusion and blindness resulted from fat injection in the nose or periorbital region,[3–5] some were reported with fat injection into the nasolabial folds[6] or even the lower lip.[7]

Obviously, artertial embolization can also affect the mucosa, conjunctiva, or skin and result in necrosis. There has been a report of blindness, stroke, and skin necrosis from the injection of only 0.5 mL of filler into the left side of the nasal bridge.[8] Even a small amount injected into the lower face has been reported as having devastating complications; unilateral blindness and brain infarction occurred after the injection of only 0.5 mL into a nasolabial fold.[6]

How it occurs?

The retinal artery and posterior ciliary arteries are proximal branches of the ophthalmic internal carotid arteries. If the opening to the needle is in the lumen of an artery, the filler will be injected into the lumen of the cannulated artery. As more pressure is applied to the plunger, the filler displaces the arterial blood and travels as a column proximally past the origin of the retinal artery. A tiny amount of the filler slipping into the retinal artery can precipitate a central retinal artery blockage, usually resulting in permanent blindness. It is also possible to force the column back into the internal carotid artery and embolize into any area supplied by the internal carotid area, and this may result in a stroke.

How to avoid?

To avoid such complications, do not use sharp needles. Additionally, one should limit bolus size, limit syringe size (only 1 mL syringe to the face), and avoid using ratcheting guns. Small and sharp needles/cannulas are much more likely to perforate the wall of an artery and cannulate the artery lumen than are the larger, blunter instruments. Therefore, extreme caution should be taken when sharp needles of any type are used to inject particulate matter into the face.

The volume placed with each pass of the cannula should also be limited. Infiltration of less than 0.1 mL with each pass of the cannula is recommended in the face. To be especially safe, aliquots of less than 0.033 or 0.02 mL are preferable in the periorbital region. Additionally, a vasoconstricted artery is harder to cannulate than a vasodilated one, so epinephrine should be considered for use at the injection site for the placement of fillers. When using a larger syringe (10 or 20 mL) for infiltration of the fat, the surgeon's control over the volume injected is less than with the smaller syringe, so it is easier to mistakenly inject a larger amount or to inject with a high pressure. Thus, it is strongly recommended to use only 1 mL Luer-Lok syringes for subcutaneous infiltration into the face. Blindness has also occurred following soft tissue injections with assistive mechanical devices that may create strong pressures during the injection of soft tissues.

Fat Necrosis: Calcifications and Oil Cysts

Necrosis of grafted fat tissue induces cicatrization, calcifications, and oil cysts if the necrosis size is substantial. Although a single dead adipocyte (50–150 µ) can be completely absorbed, significant numbers of oil drops are replaced with collagen matrix (cicatrization).[9] If the cicatrization has a central tiny oil drop (<1 mm), chronic inflammation persists and a sand-like macrocalcification (0.3–2 mm) can develop over the first 5 years. In the event that the fat necrosis is large in size (>10 mm), the necrotic tissue becomes an oil cyst within 6 to 12 months after grafting, which presents never-ending inflammation. Oil cysts are permanently problematic; they neither become silent, nor reduced in size.[1]

Oil cysts can occur after roughly performed fat injection and are more likely to be seen after large-volume fat grafting such as the breast and buttock. It should be noted that the well-projected breast and buttock with a tight skin envelop are uncommon outcomes after fat grafting (common after synthetic implant placement) and can result from oil cyst formation (**Fig. 1**).

How it occurs?

Dead adipocytes become oil droplets and are first surrounded by infiltrated M1-type (inflammatory) macrophages for phagocytosis.[9] The absorption of oil is a very slow process; it takes weeks for a 1 mm oil droplet to be completely absorbed. At a later stage, stratified layers of M2-type (anti-inflammatory) macrophages surround the M1 macrophages and form a fibrous cyst wall. The formation of cyst wall stops the oil absorption process, and the size of oil cysts will not change any later than 1 year after surgery, although the calcification process of the cyst wall continues to progress over several years due to the persisting inflammation.[1]

How to avoid?

Recent findings on the mechanism of fat graft survival and regeneration suggested that fat particles with a more than 2 to 3 mm diameter cannot be engrafted at 100%. Fat necrosis after grafting largely depends on the injection technique/volume and microenvironments of the recipient site. If one

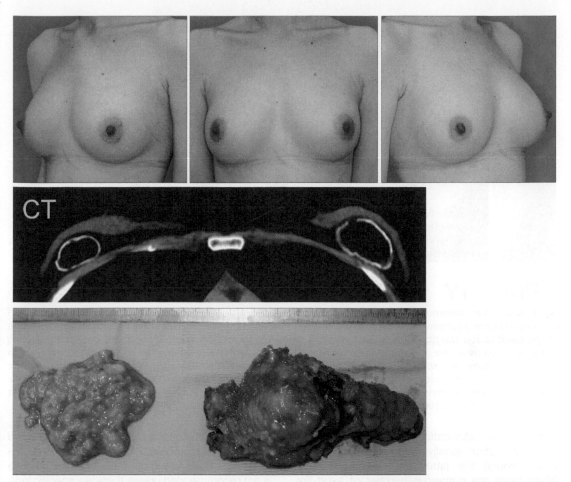

Fig. 1. A case of oil cysts. A 24-year-old woman underwent fat grafting for cosmetic breast augmentation 2 years earlier. She recognized hardness of the entire breast at 6 months and gradually recognized tenderness and abnormal sensations. (*Top*) She had well-projected breasts with tight skin. The contour of the upper pole looked similar to a breast with implant contracture. (*Middle*) Preoperative computed tomography (CT) scan showed that there was a single large calcified oil cyst under each mammary gland. It was suspected that 100 to 200 mL of fat tissue had been introduced in a bolus injection before. (*Bottom*) Removed oil cysts were filled with muddy content caused by fat necrosis. The oil cyst wall had innermost and outermost fibrous layers. (*Adapted from* Mineda K, Kuno S, Kato H, et al. Chronic inflammation and progressive calcification as a result of fat necrosis: the worst outcome in fat grafting. Plast Reconstr Surg 2014;133:1064–72; with permission.)

wants to make a fat column (noodle) with 2 or 3 mm diameter, 1 mL fat has theoretically to be a noodle of 32 or 14 cm long, respectively. Such a careful and meticulous injection technique is critical to avoid a large fat necrosis forming an oil cyst. One needs to use smaller injection syringes such as 1 mL syringe for the face and 3 mL syringe for the body. Special injection syringes/devices may be helpful if they facilitate a controllable precise infiltration of fat tissue.

How to treat?
Once an oil cyst is established, never-ending inflammation and progressive calcification of the cystic wall can induce symptoms such as hard lumps, tenderness/pain, abnormal/heating sensation, contracture, projected breast with tight skin envelop, and/or general fatigue. It is not easy to treat the oil cyst and its associated symptoms without surgical resection. Another option is to partially cut the cystic wall with an 14–18G needle and squeeze it, leading to leakage and phagocytosis of oil or necrotic tissue.

Calcifications in mammogram
Small fat necrosis induces a fibrous deposit, which later develops into a sand-like micro/macro-calcification over years (**Fig. 2**), whereas large fat necrosis induces an oil cyst, of which fibrous wall will be calcified over time and present an

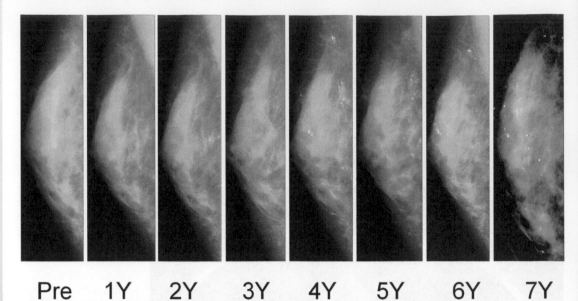

Pre   1Y   2Y   3Y   4Y   5Y   6Y   7Y

Fig. 2. Sequential mammography images of a case with fat grafting to the breast. Mammograms were taken sequentially from a patient (30-year-old woman) who underwent fat grafting to the breast with no postoperative lumps. Calcification was not apparent at 1 year, but sand-like macrocalcifications were clearly detected at 2 years and progressed over time, indicating that calcifications grow progressively at least up to several years even with no noticeable lump. It is suspected that small necrotic areas become sand-like calcifications, while larger necrotic areas becomes oil cysts with eggshell-like calcification. (*Adapted from* Mineda K, Kuno S, Kato H, et al. Chronic inflammation and progressive calcification as a result of fat necrosis: the worst outcome in fat grafting. Plast Reconstr Surg 2014;133:1064–72; with permission.)

egg-shell-like calcification (**Fig. 3**). The former-type calcification usually shows no clinical symptoms, though the latter can be troublesome. When there are numerous number of sand-like and/or egg shell-like calcifications detected in the mammogram, they interfere with detailed evaluation of mammographic images and precise diagnosis of breast cancer. Visual features of each calcification induced by fat necrosis are generally distinct and can be differentiated by professional diagnostic radiologists from those of microcalcifications by breast cancer, and therefore, it is not a problem that there are several typical sand-like macrocalcifications seen in the mammogram. Plastic surgeons should be careful not to inject fat into the mammary gland and to avoid any bolus injections. Ultrasound assessment at 1 month after lipoinjection is particularly valuable for a surgeon to detect even tiny oil drops and learn how well the injection procedure was performed.

Other Complications

Infection

Although infection is uncommon with fat grafting, infection following fat necrosis or hematoma can occur. As the grafted fat is not vascularized, it can be a focus of infection once severely contaminated by bacteria. Sterile technique should be observed at all times. Intraoperative antibiotics are recommended to use, but perioperative use of antibiotics is not recommended unless there is a specific indication. In cases of delayed infection, a high index of suspicion should be maintained for mycobacterial or other unusual infections.

Damage to underlying structures

Even a blunt cannula, when inserted for removal and placement of fat, can damage underlying structures such as nerves, muscles, glands, and blood vessels using this technique; however, permanent injuries are extremely rare.

Pneumonia

In the learning curve of fat injection to the breast, it is rare but possible to induce pneumonia. Pneumonia is induced by damaging the pleura with an injection cannula/needle. Therefore, great care should be taken to avoid when introducing fat into the bottom layer close to the rib. Pneumonia is usually first recognized as a complaint of chest pain in the next morning and can be diagnosed by monitor of oxygen saturation, chest X-ray, and/or CT scan. If pneumonia is a minor one, it can be treated by a conservative treatment such as waiting with careful monitor of X-ray and symptoms.

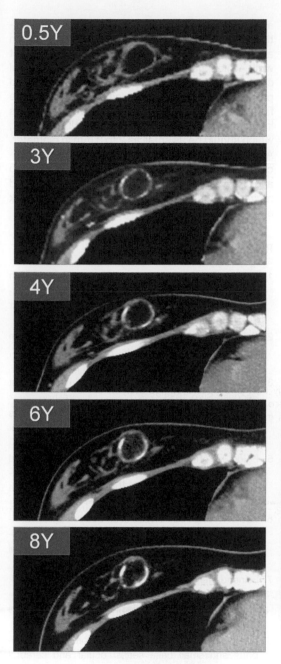

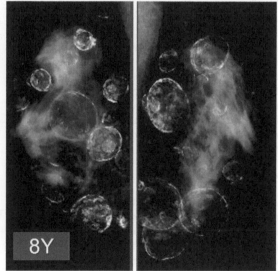

Fig. 3. Sequential CT images and mammography of oil cysts. (*Left*) CT was sequentially taken from a patient (34-year-old woman) with multiple oil cysts in both breasts who did not undergo any removal of the cysts. The size of oil cyst did not change between 3 and 8 years, but calcifications progressed during the period. (*Right*) Mammography of the same patient at 8 years. Many eggshell-like calcifications are shown. (*Modified from* Mineda K, Kuno S, Kato H, et al. Chronic inflammation and progressive calcification as a result of fat necrosis: the worst outcome in fat grafting. Plast Reconstr Surg 2014;133:1064–72.)

Aesthetic problems and complications

One of the most common complications after fat grafting is related to aesthetics, such as the placement of too much or too little fat in a specified area. The presence of irregularities, which can be caused by the intrinsic nature of the patient's body, from the technique used for placement, and from migration after placement, is also noted. Irregularities after fat grafting diminish significantly as the surgeon gains experience with the technique. In addition, the overgrowth of fat grafts can occur with weight gain. More perplexing, fat grafts can grow in people with stable weight. Such overgrowth, not related to weight gain, is most often seen in reaction to medications but can occur without apparent cause.

Swelling and downtime

One of the most difficult tasks for the surgeon is preparing patients to expect the bruising and swelling created by this technique. The placement of fatty tissue may create remarkable swelling in the recipient tissues. This depends on a number of factors, including the amount of fat placed, the anatomic location to which it is grafted, the specific technique and instruments used, medications the patient takes, and the age and genetic makeup of the patient. Patient care after fat transplantation is directed at minimizing swelling and avoiding migration. Elevation, cold therapy, and external pressure with elastic tape or Tegaderm (3M, Maplewood, MN, USA) help prevent swelling. Certain medications (*Arnica montana* and bromelain) may also speed recovery. The patient is asked to avoid heavy pressure on the grafted areas for 7 to 10 days to avoid migration of the grafted fat.

Swelling can be especially bothersome and prolonged in the periorbital region, particularly the lower eyelid. Any pigmentation in the lower lid will appear darker with bruising, which can last even in a minimal form for many weeks. A slight staining of the skin, possibly hemosiderin deposits or other pigment changes, can remain for months in some patients after minimal fat grafting to the lower eyelid.

Donor site problems

Finally, many patients find the removal of fat and the body contouring performed at the same time to be advantageous, yet even a surgeon who is facile at liposuction may produce liposuction deformities. Furthermore, some patients simply do not have adequate donor sites, especially if they have previously undergone liposuction. Complications of the donor sites are rare, but irregularity of the surface could occur, particularly when an excessive volume liposuction is performed in very thin patients.

SUMMARY

Accidental injection of soft tissue fillers into the arterial system can result in catastrophic complications. Blindness and stroke have occurred as a result of the injection of soft tissue fillers in almost every part of the face. During injection of any soft tissue filler in the face, consideration should be given to the possibility of cannulation of arteries and to the volume of filler injected at any instant. The injection of large boluses of soft tissue fillers in the face and the use of sharp needles or cannulas that can easily perforate an arterial wall should be avoided. Another major complication

after fat grafting is oil cyst formation and calcifications. Oil cysts show never-ending inflammation and progressive calcification in the cyst wall, which can induce many types of clinical complaints including unmanageable infection and pain. Oil cysts are a typical result of roughly done fat injection, and surgeons should avoid any bolus injection and introduce noodle-like columns of fat, which should be as small as 2 to 3 mm in diameter. Although fat grafting is a minimally invasive surgical procedure, surgeon have to be cautious to avoid any unexpected damage to the donor and recipient sites to minimize the perioperative risk and complications.

REFERENCES

1. Mineda K, Kuno S, Kato H, et al. Chronic inflammation and progressive calcification as a result of fat necrosis: the worst outcome in fat grafting. Plast Reconstr Surg 2014;133:1064–72.
2. Coleman SR. Avoidance of arterial occlusion from injection of soft tissue fillers. Aesthet Surg J 2002; 22:555–7.
3. Teimourian B. Blindness following fat injection. Plast Reconstr Surg 1988;82:361.
4. Dreizen NG, Framm L. Sudden unilateral visual loss after autologous fat injection into the glabellar area. Am J Ophthalmol 1989;107:85–7.
5. Egido JA, Arroyo R, Marcos A, et al. Middle cerebral artery embolism and unilateral visual loss after autologous fat injection into the glabellar area. Stroke 1993;24:615–6.
6. Lee DH, Yang HN, Kim JC, et al. Sudden unilateral visual loss and brain infraction after autologous fat injection into the nasolabial groove. Br J Ophthalmol 1996;80:1026–7.
7. Feinendegen DL, Baumgartner RW, Schroth G, et al. Middle cerebral artery occlusion and ocular fat embolism after autologous fat injection in the face. J Neurol 1998;245:53–4.
8. Danesh-Mayer HV, Savino PJ, Sergott RC. Case reports and small case series: ocular and cerebral ischemia following facial injection of autologous fat. Arch Ophthalmol 2001;19:777–8.
9. Kato H, Mineda K, Eto H, et al. Degeneration, regeneration, and cicatrization after fat grafting: dynamic total tissue remodeling during the first three months. Plast Reconstr Surg 2014;133:303e–13e.

Future Perspectives of Fat Grafting

Lee L.Q. Pu, MD, PhD[a],*, Kotaro Yoshimura, MD[b], Sydney R. Coleman, MD[c]

KEYWORDS

- Fat grafting • Soft-tissue augmentation • Soft-tissue reconstruction • Regenerative surgery
- Fat grafting research

KEY POINTS

- Future perspectives of fat grafting from 3 editors are summarized in this review. Fat grafting will continue to play an important role in cosmetic and reconstructive surgery.
- Fat grafting can be a good option to replace some of the "traditional" procedures in cosmetic and reconstructive surgery.
- Fat grafting may become a regenerative procedure that can be used to treat varieties of difficult clinical problems that have not been solved at the present time. More definitive studies are still needed in order to answer any specific questions related to fat grafting including the best technique and the role of ADSCs.

INTRODUCTION

Autologous fat grafting has become a popular procedure in both cosmetic and reconstructive plastic surgery. It has been a "hot topic" in almost all major plastic surgery meetings lately and many advances in fat grafting have been made in this exciting field of plastic surgery. Modern fat grafting started as a means for facial rejuvenation and correction for soft tissue counter deformity in the mid 1990s and championed by Coleman. It had a "bad reputation" for years, especially in the United States, as the procedure with unachievable or unpredictable outcome and uncertain safety.[1] However, as we learn more and more about fat grafting and its potential,[2] many reputable plastic surgeons are able to achieve good to excellent results with the procedure and to expand its role in many other areas of plastic surgery, including cosmetic and reconstructive surgery of the breast.[3] In this last article, 3 editors put together their perspective views on future autologous fat grafting.

FACIAL REJUVENATION

Autologous fat grafting will continue to play an important role in facial rejuvenation. As a matter of fact, it will, as a relatively less invasive surgical procedure, gradually replace many open approaches to early or even moderately facial aging.[4] It will also expand its role in combination with a traditional face lift surgery especially for correction of facial aging in the central portion of the face such as in the lid/cheek junction, tear trough, nasolabial fold, or perioral region because these areas are typically not corrected by a traditional face lift; fat grafting will likely achieve permanent improvement when comparing with a synthetic filler such as hyaluronic acid for the same purpose. Because of the unique regenerative potential of fat, presumably because of the potential effect of adipose derived stem cells, it has a unique feature not only to correct soft tissue deficiency but also to rejuvenate the skin of the face.[5] It is quite likely that fat grafting will play a more important role in facial rejuvenation and only stromal vascular fraction (SVF) other than fat will be injected for facial

[a] Division of Plastic Surgery, University of California, Davis, 2221 Stockton Boulevard, Suite 2123, Sacramento, CA 95817, USA; [b] Department of Plastic Surgery, School of Medicine, University of Tokyo, 7-3-1 Hongo, Bunkyo-ku, Tokyo 113-8655, Japan; [c] Department of Plastic Surgery, New York University Langone Medical Center, New York, NY, USA
* Corresponding author.
E-mail address: lee.pu@ucdmc.ucdavis.edu

Clin Plastic Surg 42 (2015) 389–394
http://dx.doi.org/10.1016/j.cps.2015.03.007
0094-1298/15/$ – see front matter © 2015 Elsevier Inc. All rights reserved.

rejuvenation because of the regenerative potential of adipose derived stem cells within SVF. As surgeons gain more clinical experience and follow their patients for longer term, better results can be achieved by fat grafting in combination with a traditional open procedure for facial rejuvenation than that by an open face lift surgery alone.[6] It can also be true that fat grafting will replace some of traditional rhinoplasty procedures because it could improve the contour of the nose.[7]

CRANIOFACIAL DEFORMITY

Fat grafting is also going to play an increased role for correction of craniofacial deformities secondary to congenital deformity or traumatic injury. Fat grafting would correct soft tissue deformity and its preliminary results have been amazing.[8] It can also be an useful alternative to microvascular free tissue transfer to the face with a significant soft tissue deformity.[9] Fat grafting in combination with a traditional bony craniofacial reconstruction will provide the patient with much better clinical outcome than a traditional craniofacial approach with primary emphasis on bony reconstruction. In addition, the regenerative potential of adipose tissue cannot be replaced by any traditional craniofacial surgical approach in the head and neck region.[10] The regenerative nature of fat has been applied innovatively by our ENT colleagues to treat various vocal cord pathologies with good success and minimal or no serious complications.[11] Fat grafting as primary or adjunct procedure will be widely performed for management of many craniofacial pathologies.

COSMETIC AND RECONSTRUCTIVE BREAST SURGERY

The role of fat grafting in cosmetic and reconstructive breast surgery will continue to evolve. It will continue to become a widely used adjunctive procedure to improve the clinical outcome of both cosmetic and reconstructive breast surgery. Fat grafting for primary or secondary breast augmentation will be a common procedure of choice for both patients and plastic surgeons. Fat grafting will become a valid option for correction of lumpectomy defect for treatment of early breast cancer. In addition, fat grafting for total breast reconstruction after mastectomy may become a clinical reality and achieve the clinical outcome and patient satisfaction that cannot be achieved with an implant or flap surgery. The future of fat grafting in cosmetic and reconstructive breast surgery can be further classified into 4 major areas: breast augmentation, breast enhancement, correction of breast asymmetry and congenital deformity, and breast reconstruction.

Breast Augmentation

Although fat grafting for primary breast augmentation had a "bad reputation" in the past, the procedure itself has gained more popularity recently and is being performed more and more by plastic surgeons worldwide for primary breast augmentation.[1,3] There are adequate studies in the literature to support the efficacy and safety of fat grafting for primary breast augmentation.[12–14] Although there is lack of standardized technique for fat grafting to the breast, plastic surgeons have improved their surgical technique of fat grafting for primary breast augmentation so that satisfactory results can be achieved in selective patients and there is no need for an implant-based breast augmentation.[15,16] More study needs to be conducted to further confirm the efficacy and safety of fat grafting as a primary means for breast augmentation. In addition, surgical techniques also need to be standardized to avoid complications and shorten the learning curve in fat grafting for primary breast augmentation.

Breast Enhancement

Fat grafting, as a valid option, will be used widely in conjunction with traditional mastopexy or implant exchange to achieve a better outcome in aesthetic breast surgery.[17,18] It provides another option to manage "soft tissue deficiency" for selected patients. In addition, the concept of composite breast augmentation with implant and fat grafting has been introduced, which may provide clinical outcome in breast augmentation for selected patients that cannot be achieved by either option alone.[19]

Correction of Breast Asymmetry and Congenital Deformity

Fat grafting as a popular procedure will probably replace most of the current techniques for correction of breast asymmetry.[20] This might be true for correction of some less significant breast asymmetries. Breast augmentation with implant, mastopexy, or breast reduction will continue to play a role for the correction of significant breast asymmetry. Fat grafting itself will become a primary option for correction of several breast congenital deformities, such as the Poland syndrome or tuberous breast. It will likely correct those congenital deformities without the need for a traditional breast implant or flap reconstruction.[21]

Breast Reconstruction

Fat grafting as a valid procedure will continue to be widely used in reconstructive breast surgery for a final touch up procedure after implant or flap reconstruction.[22] It has proven its role in correction of soft tissue contour deformity related to implant-based breast reconstruction.[23] Multiple fat grafts followed by implant reconstruction has its unique value after total mastectomy with irradiation therapy because the quality of irradiated skin over the implant can be improved with fat grafting.[24,25] Fat grafting will become an effective and valid option for correction of lumpectomy or even partial mastectomy defect with radiation after conservative breast surgery for treatment of early breast cancer if such an approach can be proved to be safe with no issues on future breast cancer recurrence and detection. It can potentially revolutionize the surgical approach to what used to be an "uncorrectable" clinical condition in breast reconstructive surgery. With efficacy and safety of Brava continue to be firmed, mega volume autologous fat grafting may become a clinical reality for total breast reconstruction after mastectomy without radiation and replace the traditional approach to breast reconstruction with an implant or a surgical flap for breast reconstruction, although multiple sessions are needed.[26–28] However, a standardized technique for mega volume fat grafting needs to be established, just like an implant-based reconstruction or autologous flap-based breast reconstruction, so that the technique of mega volume fat grafting can be learned by most plastic surgeons to produce a consistent, if not better, clinical outcomes in total breast reconstruction for patients after mastectomy.

GLUTEAL AUGMENTATION

An implant-based gluteal augmentation has been adapted primarily by Brazilian plastic surgeons and an optimal outcome can be achieved with intramuscular placement of a gluteal implant.[29] Autologous fat grafting for gluteal augmentation has continued to evolve and recent experience from worldwide plastic surgeons has been good. Because fat grafting involves the harvest of fat from many unwanted areas in patients, fat grafting for gluteal augmentation will continue to be a popular and desirable approach to body contour surgery, requested by patients. With an improvement in standardized technique of fat grafting, fat grafting will play a more important role in gluteal augmentation and may replace implant-based gluteal augmentation if the patient has a great enough amount of fat as donor materials.[30,31]

HAND REJUVENATION

As hand rejuvenation becomes a demanding procedure for certain kind of patients, autologous fat grafting will continue to be safe and effective procedure for hand rejuvenation.[32] Because fat may not only serve as filler, but also has the regenerative potential to improve the quality of soft tissue and skin on the dorsal side of the hands, fat grafting can be an attractive procedure for hand rejuvenation and achieve better outcomes in the hand after fat grafting that cannot be accomplished by any other means, because synthetic fillers such as hyaluronic acid work poorly for hand rejuvenation and fat is definitively better filler to be used for such a clinical application.[4]

REGENERATIVE SURGERY

Autologous fat grafting has been used by some investigators to treat difficult wounds that have failed the conventional wound therapy.[33,34] Although the exact mechanism still remains unknown, most investigators believe the ability of fat grafting to heal the difficult wound would at least partially owing to the regenerative potential of adipose derived stem cells within the fat grafts.[33] If this concept can be confirmed in future studies, fat grafting will have an expanded role in reconstructive surgery to improve healing of difficult wounds and may replace some of the traditional surgical procedures, such as a flap reconstruction or skin grafting to facilitate wound closure. In addition, its regenerative effects can improve much functionality of the involved tissues such as elasticity, vascularity, pain release, reduced inflammation, and a lesser degree of immunoreaction. These effects, in general, cannot be achieved by any of "traditional" procedures in plastic surgery. This can be true when percutaneous aponeurotomy and lipofilling are performed to treat scar contracture as a regenerative alternative to a flap reconstruction.[35] This kind of new surgical approach is minimally invasive and "incisionless"; only needles, cannulas, and syringes are used for the procedure. It may revolutionize what we do now as reconstructive plastic surgeons because of the regenerative potential of fat grafting.

One of the great examples is that fat grafting can be performed after extensive percutaneous aponeurotomy for treatment of Dupuytren's contracture and fat grafts as lipofiller are placed between the skin and underlying structures of the finger and hand to lead to scarless supple skin and better functional outcome of the finger or hand.[36] It is possible that most patients with less severe Dupuytren's contracture can be treated with this new minimally invasive procedure once plastic surgeons have mastered their technique of percutaneous aponeurotomy and fat grafting.

Fat grafting may also be performed to the hand of patients with Raynaud phenomenon to reduce pain, cold attacks, and ulcerations, and to improve skin, soft tissue texture, and hand function. Several beneficial effects after fat grafting in this group of patients may be the contribution of adipose-derived stem cells, but the true mechanism of stem cells on ischemic tissue remains hypothetical.[37] However, fat grafting as a safe and well-recognized procedure provides a new alternative and potentially regenerative approach to this difficult clinical problem and may be used more often in the future.

Fat grafting will continually be performed to improve the appearance of scars, especially in the head and neck.[38,39] Once again, the observed effects of fat on scars are contributed mainly by adipose derived stem cells. Thus, fat grafting can be a new alternative for treatment of scars in selected patients with promising results and future potential.

Fat grafting, as an established procedure, has been performed for treatment of scar contracture induced pain in patients with "postmastectomy pain syndrome." The measurable improvements are partially attributed to scar remodeling through new collagen deposition, local hypervascularity, and dermal hyperplasia.[40] The regenerative role of fat in scarred areas is thought to be the result of releases of multiple nerve entrapments so that neuropathic pain is improved. In addition, the improvement in neurogenic pain may be maintained by placing fat grafts around the nerve to avoid the recurrence of scar contracture. Importantly, a well-conducted experimental study demonstrated that fat grafting can alleviate burn-induced neuropathic pain in rats.[41] If the efficacy and safety of fat grafting for treatment of neuropathic pain syndrome can be confirmed in future studies, this relatively simple approach will provide a new solution for this clinical condition, a pain syndrome that relates to various scar contracture or scar fibrosis in head and neck, breasts, or hands.

As the value of the SVF is recognized, SVF in combination with conventional fat grafting has been used clinically for improvement of the results in facial rejuvenation and primary breast augmentation with an approved success.[8,42] A level I clinical trial published in *Lancet* has clearly demonstrated the value of SVF to improve the survival of autologous fat grafting.[43] In addition, either non-cultured or cultured SVF has been used by investigators to treat difficult wounds, arthritis, Crohn's disease with some amazing observed results. However, concerns about the use of "collagenase" during the isolation of SVF from lipoaspirates has been raised in the United States, which precludes the immediate clinical application of SVF-enriched fat grafting in patients. Nanofat grafting, as a possible alternative, has recently been described to obtain SVF-like cellular components without collagenase. It employs intense mechanical shearing to rupture adipocytes, leaving a nanofat sample that is rich in stem cell content. It has proven clinical efficacy in facial rejuvenation; however, the exact constituents and regenerative potential of this mix has yet to be defined.[44] In addition, SVF may be processed without the need of collagenase.[45] If the efficacy of this technique can be confirmed by future study, SVF-enriched fat grafting or SVF alone can be performed clinically for various conditions with potential better outcome.

RESEARCH IN FAT GRAFTING

It remains true that many questions need to be answered in fat grafting, for example, fat harvest, processing, and placement, preparation of the recipient site, and the role of stem cells.[46] We shall see more and more studies specifically designed to answer these questions related to fat grafting in the future because there are an increased number of publications in this exciting flied. We shall have better understanding of the mechanism how fat grafts survive; for example, the graft survival theory versus the host replacement theory or both.[47,48] Although we are just starting to realize the role of adipose-derived stem cells in autologous fat grafting, more definitive studies are needed to better elucidate the role of adipose derived stem cells in fat grafting. Expanding knowledge of adipose-derived stem cells would allow a more effective way to use SVFs for treatment of difficult clinical problems that have not been solved at the present time. In addition, cryopreservation of fat or adipose-derived stem cells may also explore possible future application of fat grafting because no additional harvest of fat grafts are needed and potentially cryopreserved SVF may provide younger adipose-derived stem cells from the same patient.[49]

STANDARDIZED TECHNIQUE IN FAT GRAFTING

Plastic surgeons will continue to refine their technique in fat grafting, but more important to standardize the technique for fat grafting probably based on the volume needed for their patients.[13] For example, small volume (<100 mL) fat grafting for facial rejuvenation or other regenerative approach, large volume (100–200 mL) for correction of significant contour deformities after breast augmentation or reconstruction and mega volume (>200 mL) fat grafting for primary breast augmentation, breast reconstruction, and gluteal augmentation. Clinically, certain type of surgical instruments or equipment also need to be studied so that plastic surgeons will use better and more reliable instruments or equipment to perform small, large or mega volume fat grafting for their patients.

SUMMARY

Autologous fat grafting is an exciting field in plastic and reconstructive surgery. Fat serves as a filler as well as its role for tissue regeneration will likely play a more important role in our specialty. As we learn more about the basic science of fat grafting and the standardized techniques and instruments used for fat grafting, this procedure alone or in conjunction with some less invasive procedures may be able to replace many operations that we perform currently. The minimally invasive nature of the procedure will benefit greatly our cosmetic and reconstructive patients, and may even achieve better clinical outcomes. We live in this exciting time of plastic surgery and look forward to the new era of our specialty.

REFERENCES

1. Gutowski KA, ASPS Fat Graft Task Force. Current applications and safety of autologous fat grafts: a report of the ASPS fat graft task force. Plast Reconstr Surg 2009;124:272–80.
2. Gir P, Brown SA, Oni G, et al. Fat grafting: evidence-based review on autologous fat harvesting, processing, reinjection, and storage. Plast Reconstr Surg 2012;130:249–58.
3. Kling RE, Mehrara BJ, Pusic AL, et al. Trends in autologous fat grafting to the breast: a national survey of the American Society of Plastic Surgeons. Plast Reconstr Surg 2013;132:35–46.
4. Coleman SR. Structural fat grafting: more than a permanent filler. Plast Reconstr Surg 2006;118:108S–20S.
5. Mojallal A, Lequeux C, Shipkov C, et al. Improvement of skin quality after fat grating: clinical observation and an animal study. Plast Reconstr Surg 2009;124:765–74.
6. Rohrich RJ, Ghavami A, Constantine FC, et al. Lift-and-fill face lift: integrating the fat compartments. Plast Reconstr Surg 2014;133:756o 67o.
7. Erol OO. Microfat grafting in nasal surgery. Aesthet Surg J 2013;34:671–86.
8. Tanikawa DY, Aguena M, Bueno DF, et al. Fat grafts supplemented with adipose-derived stromal cells in the rehabilitation of patients with craniofacial microsomia. Plast Reconstr Surg 2013;132:141–52.

9. Tanna N, Wan DC, Kawamoto HK, et al. Craniofacial microsomia soft-tissue reconstruction comparison: inframammary extended circumflex scapular flap versus serial fat grafting. Plast Reconstr Surg 2011;127:802–11.
10. Phulpin B, Gangloff P, Tran N, et al. Rehabilitation of irradiated head and neck tissues by autologous fat transplantation. Plast Reconstr Surg 2013;132:141–52.
11. DeFatta RA, DeFatta RJ, Sataloff RT. Laryngeal lipotransfer: review of a 14-year experience. J Voice 2013;27:512–5.
12. Coleman SR, Saboeiro AP. Fat grafting to the breast revisited: safety and efficacy. Plast Reconstr Surg 2007;119:775–85.
13. Del Vecchio DA, Bucky LP. Breast augmentation using preexpansion and autologous fat transplantation: a clinical radiographic study. Plast Reconstr Surg 2011;127:2241–450.
14. Veber M, Tourasse C, Toussoun G, et al. Radiographic findings after breast augmentation by autologous fat transfer. Plast Reconstr Surg 2011;127:1289–99.
15. Khouri RK, Rigotti G, Cardoso E, et al. Megavolume autologous fat transfer: part I. Theory and principles. Plast Reconstr Surg 2014;133:550–7.
16. Khouri RK, Rigotti G, Cardoso E, et al. Megavolume autologous fat transfer: part II. Practice and techniques. Plast Reconstr Surg 2014;133:1369–77.
17. Khoobehi K, Sadeghi A. Single staged mastopexy with autologous fat grafting [Abstract]. Plast Reconstr Surg 2009;124(Suppl 4):8–9.
18. Del Vecchio DA. "SIEF" – Simultaneous implant exchange with fat: a new option in revision breast implant surgery. Plast Reconstr Surg 2012;130:1187–96.
19. Auclair E, Blondeel P, Alexander D, et al. Composite breast augmentation: soft-tissue planning using implants and fat. Plast Reconstr Surg 2013;132:558–68.
20. Delay E, Sinna R, Ho Quoc C. Tuberous breast correction by fat grafting. Aesthet Surg J 2012;33:522–8.
21. Ho Quoc C, Sinna R, Gourari A, et al. Percutaneous fasciotomies and fat grafting: indication for breast surgery. Aesthet Surg J 2013;34:671–86.
22. Kanchwala S, Glatt BS, Conant EF, et al. Autologous fat grafting to the reconstructed breast: the management of acquired contour deformities. Plast Reconstr Surg 2009;124:409–18.
23. Seth AK, Hirsch EM, Kim JY, et al. Long-term outcomes following fat grafting in prosthetic breast reconstruction: a comparative analysis. Plast Reconstr Surg 2012;130:984–90.
24. Serra-Renom JM, Munoz-Olmo JL, Serra-Mestre JM. Fat grafting in postmastectomy breast reconstruction with expanders and prostheses in patients who have received radiotherapy: formation of new

subcutaneous tissue. Plast Reconstr Surg 2010;125: 12–8.

25. Salgarello M, Visconti G, Barone-Adesi L. Fat grafting and breast reconstruction with implant: another option for irradiated breast cancer patients. Plast Reconstr Surg 2010;129:317–29.

26. Khouri RK, Eisenmann-Klein M, Cardoso E, et al. Brava and autologous fat transfer is a safe and effective breast augmentation alternative: results of a 6-year, 81-patient, prospective multicenter study. Plast Reconstr Surg 2012;129:1173–87.

27. Uda H, Sugawara Y, Sarukawa S, et al. Brava and autologous fat grafting for breast reconstruction after cancer surgery. Plast Reconstr Surg 2014;133:203–13.

28. Khouri RK, Rigotti G, Khouri RK Jr, et al. Total breast reconstruction with autologous fat transfer: review of a seven-year multicenter experience. Plast Reconstr Surg 2014;134:84–5.

29. Serra F, Aboudib JH. Gluteal implant displacement: diagnosis and treatment. Plast Reconstr Surg 2014;134:647–54.

30. Murillo WL. Buttock augmentation: case studies of fat injection monitored by magnetic resonance imaging. Plast Reconstr Surg 2004;114:1606–14.

31. Cardenas-Camarena L, Arenas-Quintana R, Robles-Cervantes JA. Buttocks fat grafting: 14 years of evolution and experience. Plast Reconstr Surg 2011; 128:545–55.

32. Coleman SR. Hand rejuvenation with structural fat grafting. Plast Reconstr Surg 2002;110:1731–44.

33. Rigotti G, Marchi A, Galie M, et al. Clinical treatment of radiotherapy tissue damage by lipoaspirate transplant: a healing process mediated by adipose-derived adult stem cells. Plast Reconstr Surg 2007;119:1409–22.

34. Del Vecchio D, Rohrich RJ. A classification of clinical fat grafting: different problems, different solutions. Plast Reconstr Surg 2012;130:511–22.

35. Khouri RK, Smit JM, Cardoso E, et al. Percutaneous aponeurotomy and lipofilling: a regenerative alternative to flap reconstruction? Plast Reconstr Surg 2013;132:1280–90.

36. Hovius SE, Kan HJ, Smit X, et al. Extensive percutaneous aponeurotomy and lipografting: a new treatment for Dupuytren disease. Plast Reconstr Surg 2011;128:221–8.

37. Bank J, Fuller SM, Henry GI, et al. Fat grafting to the hand in patients with Raynaud phenomenon: a novel

therapeutic modality. Plast Reconstr Surg 2013;133: 1109–18.

38. Mazzola IC, Cantarella G, Mazzola RF. Management of tracheostomy scar by autologous fat transplantation: a minimally invasive new approach. J Craniofac Surg 2013;24:1361–4.

39. Pallua N, Baroncini A, Alharbi Z, et al. Improvement of facial scar appearance and microcirculation by autologous lipofilling. J Plast Reconstr Aesthet Surg 2014;67:1033–7.

40. Caviggioli F, Maione L, Forcellini D, et al. Autologous fat graft in postmastectomy pain syndrome. Plast Reconstr Surg 2011;128:349–52.

41. Huang SH, Wu SH, Chang KP, et al. Autologous fat grafting alleviates burn-induced neuropathic pain in rats. Plast Reconstr Surg 2014;133:1396–405.

42. Yoshimura K, Sato K, Aoi N, et al. Cell-assisted lipotransfer for cosmetic breast augmentation: supportive use of adipose-derived stem/stromal cells. Aesthetic Plast Surg 2008;32:48–55.

43. Kolle SF, Fischer-Nielsen A, Mathiasen AB, et al. Enrichment of autologous fat grafts with ex-vivo expanded adipose tissue-derived stem cells for graft survival: a randomized placebo-controlled trial. Lancet 2013;382:1113–20.

44. Tonnard P, Verpaele A, Geert Peeters G, et al. Nanofat grafting: basic research and clinical applications. Plast Reconstr Surg 2013;132:1017–26.

45. Raposio E, Caruana G, Bonomini S, et al. Novel and effective strategy for the isolation of adipose-derived stem cells: minimally manipulated adipose- derived stem cells for more rapid and safe stem cell therapy. Plast Reconstr Surg 2014;133:1406–9.

46. Longaker MT, Aston SJ, Baker DC, et al. Fat transfer in 2014: what we do not know. Plast Reconstr Surg 2014;133:1305–7.

47. Zhao J, Yi C, Li L, et al. Observations on the survival and neovascularization of fat grafts interchanged between C57BL/6-gfp and C57BL/6 mice. Plast Reconstr Surg 2012;133:398e–406e.

48. Eto H, Kato H, Suga H, et al. The fate of adipocytes after nonvascularized fat grafting: evidence of early death and replacement of adipocytes. Plast Reconstr Surg 2012;129:1081–92.

49. Pu LL. Cryoperservation of adipose tissue. Organogenesis 2009;5:138–42.

Index

Note: Page numbers of article titles are in **boldface** type.

Clin Plastic Surg 42 (2015) 395–397
http://dx.doi.org/10.1016/S0094-1298(15)00050-4
0094-1298/15/$ – see front matter © 2015 Elsevier Inc. All rights reserved.

Moving?

Make sure your subscription moves with you!

To notify us of your new address, find your **Clinics Account Number** (located on your mailing label above your name), and contact customer service at:

Email: journalscustomerservice-usa@elsevier.com

800-654-2452 (subscribers in the U.S. & Canada)
314-447-8871 (subscribers outside of the U.S. & Canada)

Fax number: 314-447-8029

Elsevier Health Sciences Division
Subscription Customer Service
3251 Riverport Lane
Maryland Heights, MO 63043

*To ensure uninterrupted delivery of your subscription, please notify us at least 4 weeks in advance of move.

Printed and bound by CPI Group (UK) Ltd, Croydon, CR0 4YY

03/10/2024

01040376-0008